KARATEDO ARTICLES

(1913~1951)

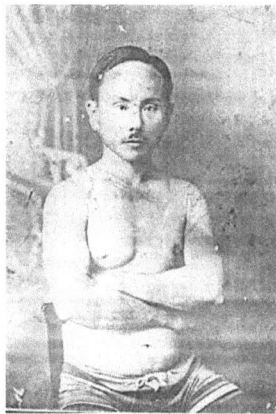

FUNAKOSHI GICHIN
TRANSLATED BY ERIC SHAHAN

Table of Contents

薩遊紀行 Record of A Journey to Satsuma Domain 1801

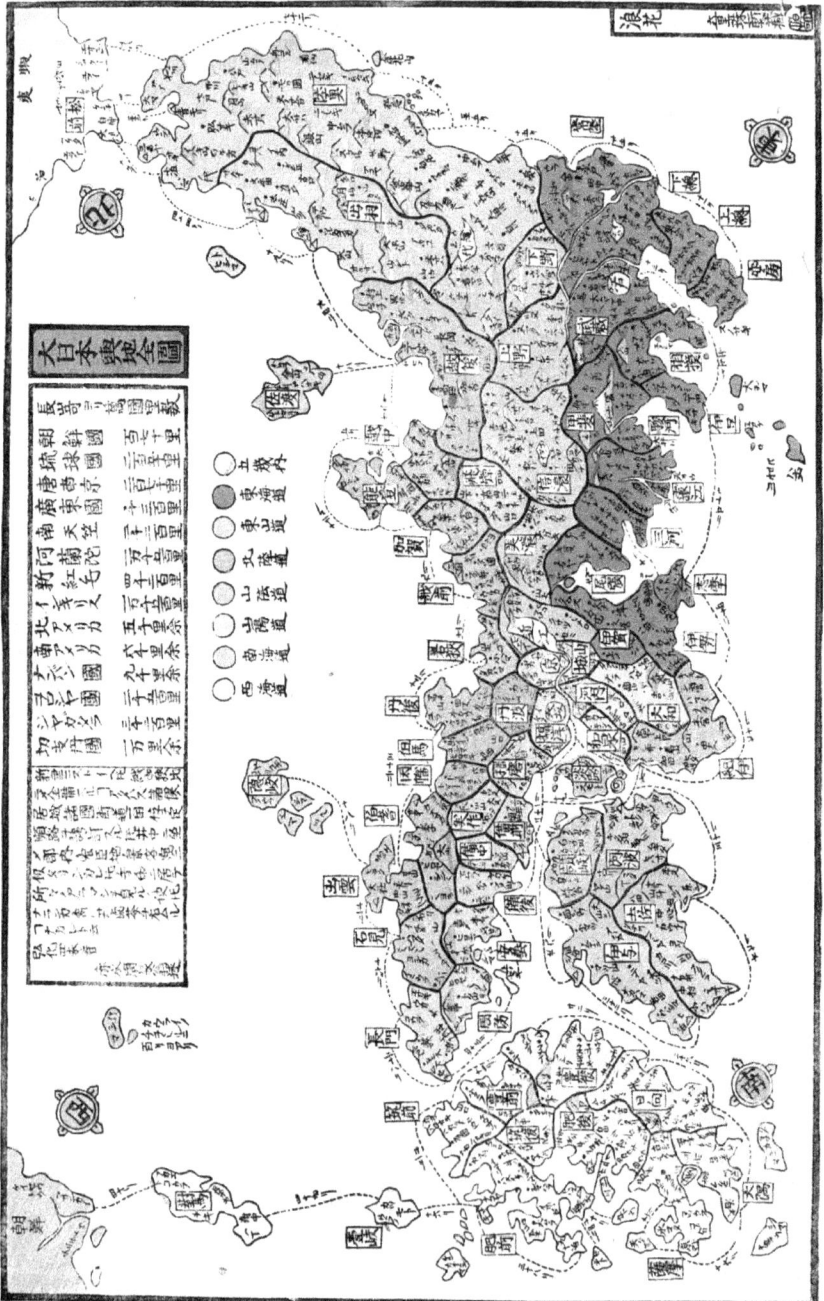

薩遊紀行 Record of A Journey to Satsuma Domain 1801

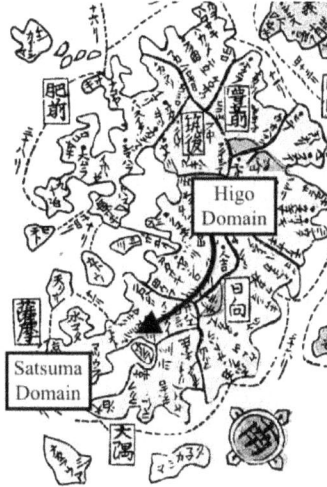

In 1801 anonymous Samurai from Higo Domain set off from Kumamoto Castle and travelled to southern Kyushu, he recorded his experiences in *Record of A Journey to Satsuma Domain*. Along the way he met a Samurai from Satsuma Domain named Mizuhara Kumajiro. Mizuhara had been stationed in Naha twice as a Samurai police officer. Each term of duty lasted three years. He described Ryukyu martial arts as follows:

> The people of Ryukyu like both Kenjutsu (swordfighting) and Yawara (Jujutsu,) but their technique is a bit amateurish. However, they have an amazing Tsukite, striking art. When training they will break anything barehanded. Their strikes could easily kill.
>
> Ryukyu people call this art Te-tsukumi, Striking in With the Hands. The Satsuma Samurai invited one practitioner to the police station. The practitioner stacked up seven roof tiles and struck them, completely obliterating six of them. If he were to strike a person it would likely rip their face off. Particularly skilled practitioners can stab with their fingers.

Karate wa Bugei no Kotsuzui nari

Karate is the Essence of Martial Arts

By Shoto

Ryukyu Shinpo Newspaper

January 9th 1913

Karate wa Bugei no Kotsuzui nari
Karate is the Essence of Martial Arts
By Shoto
Ryukyu Shinpo Newspaper
January 9th 1913

○唐手は武藝の骨髓なり

松濤

△唐手の傳來△唐手の流儀△⑴手
の種類△既往と現今△膂寒は如何
現今吾が沖繩に於て體育上唐手が柔道、劍
鑑と鼎立して盛に演せられつゝあるは蓋人

- The Introduction of Karate
- Karate Styles
- Types of Karate
- Past and Present
- What will happen in the Future?

As most people are well aware, Karate is now thriving in Okinawa as a form of physical education alongside Judo and Kendo. However, I believe the public would like to know more about when Karate began and how effective it is. Therefore, as I have spent many years training and researching Karate it would be my great pleasure to introduce what little I have learned as well as what my teachers and elders in this art have taught me.

The Introduction of Karate

The exact time when Karate was introduced to our Okinawan archipelago remains unclear, as there are no written records to confirm it, and various theories exist. However, as Dr. Iha's[1] discusses in *Biographies of Okinawan Great Men* the importation of Chinese and mainland Japanese thought likely occurred towards the end of the fourteenth century. It is thought that this occurred when the great King Sho Hashi[2] unified Sanzan, the Three Mountain Kingdoms (Middle Mountain, Southern Mountain and Northern Mountain) and restored the long-severed ties between Okinawa, Japan and China.

This can be seen as King Sho Shin[3] had ordered all the regional Daimyo to move to Shuri, thereby centralizing power. Further, all weapons were confiscated ushering in an era of peace.

However, as the people of Ryukyu had become accustomed to this prolonged peace, they suffered terribly during the Shimazu clan's *Ryukyu Seibatsu*, Conquest of Ryukyu, in 1609, the 14th year of Keicho. As the saying goes, *Just as bees have stingers and cuttlefish have ink,*[4] the people realized the necessity of remaining vigilant and prepared. The importance of *Mutekatsu Ryu Karate*, Winning Without a Weapon School of Karate, became painfully apparent. Thus, practicing Karate for self-defense became an imperative.

---

[1] Iha Fuyu 伊波普猷 (1876 ~ 1947) is considered the father of Okinawaology. Funakoshi was not only familiar with Iha's work but also interacted with him.

[2] Sho Hashi 尚巴志 (1372 ~1439)

[3] Sho Shin 尚真 (1465 ~ 1527) Sho Shin's long reign has been described as "The Great Days of Chuzan"

[4] *Hachi ni Tsurugi,Ika ni Sumijiru*
蜂に剣烏賊に墨汗
Just as bees have swords, Squid have ink. The author put the reading Hari, needle, above the Kanji for sword.

Schools of Karate

People frequently refer to the schools of Karate as Shurite, Nahate, or Tomari-te as if they were distinct styles. However, I believe that clarifying the origins of these styles will naturally dispel any confusion.

From days long past, Karate has been divided into two schools: the Shorei Ryu and the Shorin Ryu. The former emphasizes the body, while the latter emphasizes technique. The technique Waishinsan belongs to the former, and Iwaa belongs to the latter. Waishinsan refers to a burly warrior with a fat body, while Iwaa refers to a nimble warrior with a thin body who is full of vigor. The people of Naha draw on the teachings of Shorei Ryu Karate while the people in Shuri are dedicated to Shorin Ryu. The style of Karate done in Tomari is distinct as it is a blend of both Shorei and Shorin schools of Karate.

Other styles exist, such as the Shinte[5] and the rural Maikata, Dancing Style, but oral traditions indicate that the Shinte is the Tsukente[6] style, while the Maikata is unique to Okinawa.

---

[5] *Shinte* 神手 God hand style.

[6] *Tsukente* is a style of fighting with a Rokushaku Bo against a Shakusho, another name for a Sanshaku Bo.

Okinawa Traditional Kobudo 沖縄伝統古武道 1983
By Nakamoto Masahiro 仲本政博 (1938~)

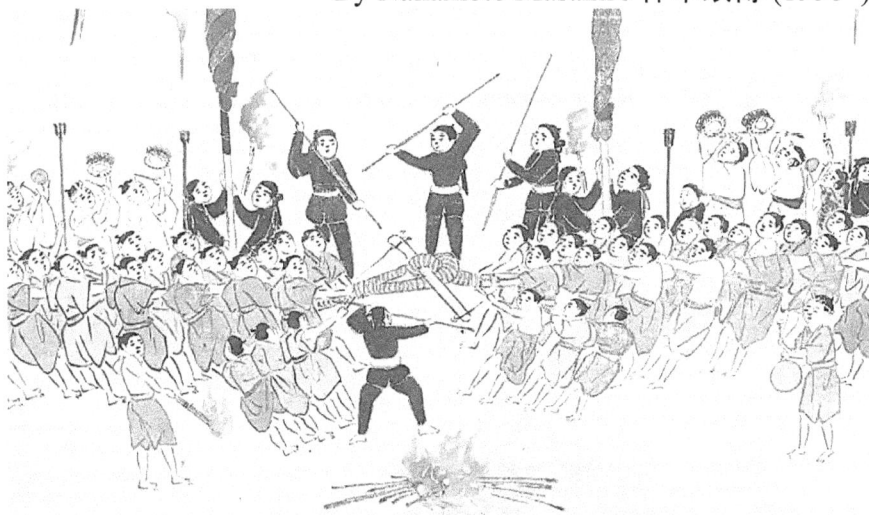

Edo Era illustration of a Bo demonstration during a tug of war.

Karate Techniques

Among the various schools mentioned above, there are over a hundred techniques. However, the techniques currently popular in Okinawa include: Sanchin, Seisan, Naihanchi, Pinan, Passai, Kuusankuu, Gojuushiho, Chintoo, Chintee, Jiin, Jitte, Wansuu, Wandoo, and Pechuurin. However, they cannot be considered to be not associated with the two previously mentioned schools.

Past and Present

In that long ago era following the Satsuma Invasion, though the fighting had ended, the effects of that tumultuous time remained. Therefore, those that trained Karate, did so in secret and made every effort prevent others from knowing what they were doing. Most practiced in closely guarded locations either in the pre-dawn hours or after the sun had set.

However, around 34th ~35th year of Meiji, 1901~1902, Karate training began to happen openly at teacher training colleges, in the same way calisthenics are taught. Every year teachers had to submit a report on the effectiveness on the program to the Ministry of Education. Today, Karate has become a topic of discussion in society, reaching even the highest levels of government. At present, the Navy Ministry is currently reviewing proposals regarding incorporating Karate. Truly a wonderous state of affairs!

What lies ahead?

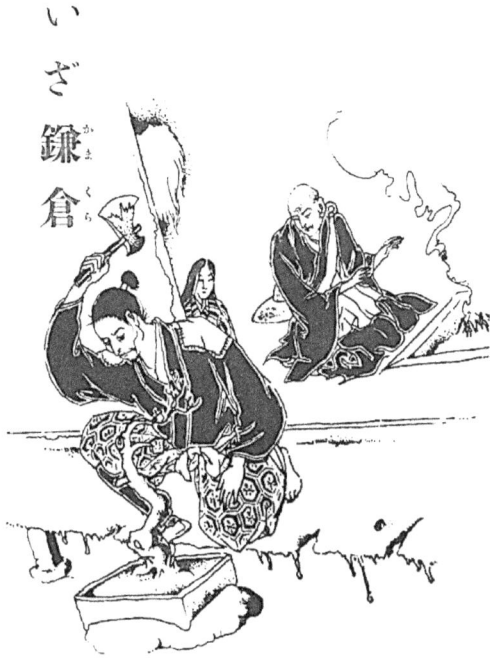

Illustration of Iza Kamakura 1926

To ensure this wonderous state of affairs continues to allow Karate flourish into the future, we must establish an organization while the great masters like Asato, Itosu and Higashionna that are still with us, and work with the prefectural authorities to formulate the best approach.[7]

The simplest strategy would be to assign graduates from the morning session who are skilled in Karate to teach in places conveniently close to them. Then do the same for graduates from the

---

[7] This article was written in 1913. Of the three Karate masters mentioned, only two were alive: Itosu Anko Itosu 糸洲安恒 (1831 ~ 1915) and Higaonna Kanryo 東恩納寛量 (1853 ~ 1915.) It is possible that Funakoshi Gichin wrote the article earlier, when Asato Anko 安里安恒 (1827 ~1906) was still alive.

evening session. [8] This would enable those interested in learning to meet frequently at convenient locations and train in their free time. This would undoubtably foster future development.

In short, every martial art has its shortcomings, meaning that you will invariably end up with some unevenness in your physical development. Yet Karate not only allows you to achieve well-rounded development it also enables you, with sufficient practice, to respond instantly and effectively should a sudden situation arise. [9]

---

[8] Classes at schools were offered in the morning and evening, called Group Two and Group Two. Group Two classes were typically for students who were working while attending school.

[9] "Should a situation suddenly arise" is *Iza Kamakura* いざ鎌倉 in Japanese. During the Kamakura period (1185~1333) if the emperor summoned the local lords, they all had to rush from their holdings to the capital Kamakura. Nowadays, the expression is used "in case that something major happens" or "event of an emergency." The origin of the phrase is as follows:

In the Kamakura era an old monk was travelling in what is now Gunma Prefecture, arrived at the house of Sano Genzaemon, a Samurai who has fallen on hard times. The monk asks to be put up for the night as there is a terrible snowstorm. While Sano used to be wealthy, his family was tricked out of their lands and all he has left are his weapons, armor and horse. He has no wood left to warm his house for his guest so he burns a treasured Bonsai tree he has growing in a pot.

The Samurai tells the priest that although he has now fallen on hard times, he will be the first to rush to his master in the event of *Iza Kamakura*, a sudden call to arms in Kamakura.

Later, the call to assemble goes out and Sano dons his armor and races to Kamakura where he is met by the monk, who turns out to be Hojo Tokiyori, who worked directly for the Shogun. Due to his loyalty, Sano's hereditary lands are restored.

As Kanna Yomori[10] said:

> *There is no beginning to the movement of Yin and Yang,*
> *and no time it is ever still*

Onga Choyu[11] took the following phrase,

> *It is not a way that can be known,*
> *for whom among men can truly know it?*

…and used "way" to compose a thirty-character poem[12] to refer to an expert in Karate:

> *To stop hidden shadowy shapelessness, use form*
> *To stop Ura, hidden, use Omote, open*
> *The true art of the warrior,*
> *lies in not being taken prisoner by Kata*

---

[10] Kanna Yomori 漢那庸森 (?~?) A Ryukyu poet.

[11] Onga Choyu 恩河朝祐 (1864~1917)

[12] The poem is not exactly thirty-one Japanese Characters, it is the name of a style of writing.

Okinawa no Bugi
The Martial Arts of Okinawa
Regarding Karate: Regarding What Asato Anko Told Me
By Shoto
Ryukyu Shinpo Newspaper
January 17th 1914

(Part 1 of 3)
The origins of Karate, Chinese Hand

Okinawa no Bugi
The Martial Arts of Okinawa
Regarding Karate: Regarding What Asato Anko Told Me
By Shoto

(Part 1 of 3)
The origins of Karate, Chinese Hand

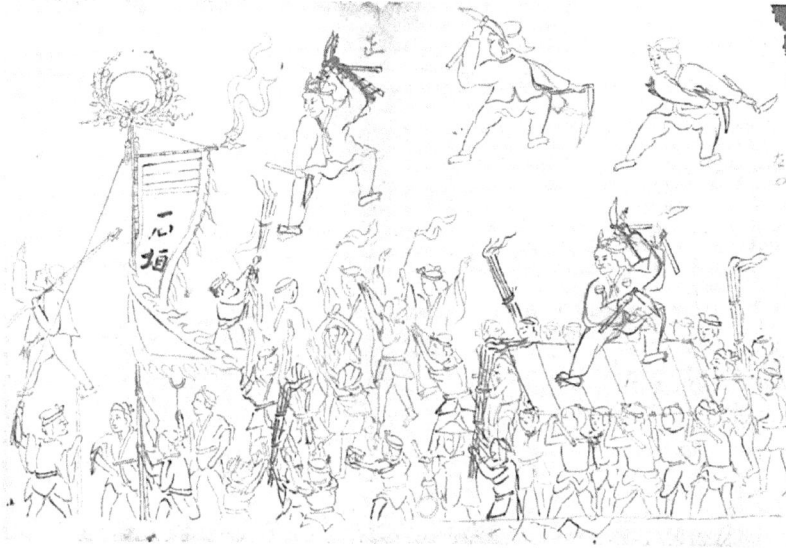

Dancers with Kama, Bo and torches
Illustration of Life In Yaeyama 八重山風俗図 Edo Era

There are many diverging theories about the origin of Karate and I am frequently asked about it. Thinking about the question now, the style of martial arts particular to Okinawa, nowadays known as Karate, originated with the Maikata dance done in the local areas and developed from there.[13]

---

[13] Maikata or Meekata is a Ryukyu traditional dance where dancers move as if doing martial arts in time with the music. It was still commonly seen up until the Second World War.

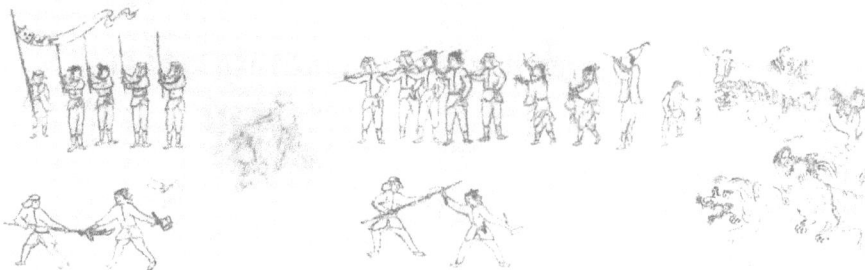

Dancers with Kama, Bo and Halberd
Illustration of Life In Yaeyama 八重山風俗図 Edo Era

You can see this in how girls grapple and fight with each other, or how boys swing their hands and strike with Tekken, iron fist, when battling each other. These ways of fighting are based on some inherited method that originated before the founding of Okinawa Prefecture, and it seems that people from Okinawa are born being able to fight that way.

Long ago, there were many famous Bushi, warriors, that taught generations of students, such as Pechin, Kyoahagon Jikki, Urasuema Yamato and Jana Uekata.[14] The style used by Akaishi of Gushikawa is based on Jana.

The name "Karate" that became known all over the world originates with a man from Akata named Todee Sakugawa.

The first person who went to Kagoshima to train Judo at government expense was Takemura of Tobara Village (Nowadays he has small house in Kamizato.) It is said that Takemura's father was a student of Todee Sakugawa so we can see that Karate was well developed in our prefecture before any Judo practitioners came to Okinawa.[15]

---

[14] Kyoahagon Jikki   京阿波根実基   (?~?)

    Urasuema Yamato   浦添真山戸   (?~?)

    Jana Uekata   謝名親方   (1549~1611)

[15] Judo was created in 1882.

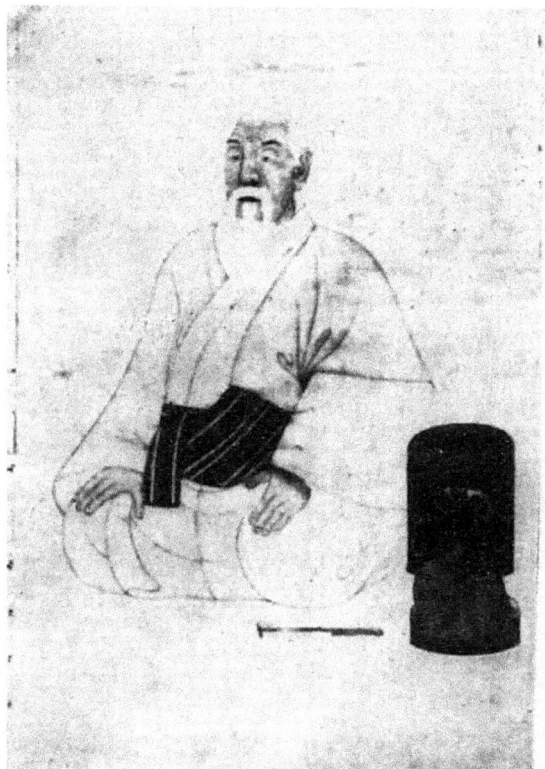

盛島親方の肖像

Portrait of Morishima
孤島苦の琉球史
Okinawa History: Struggles on a Lonely Island
Iha Fuyu 伊波普猷 1876-1947
1926

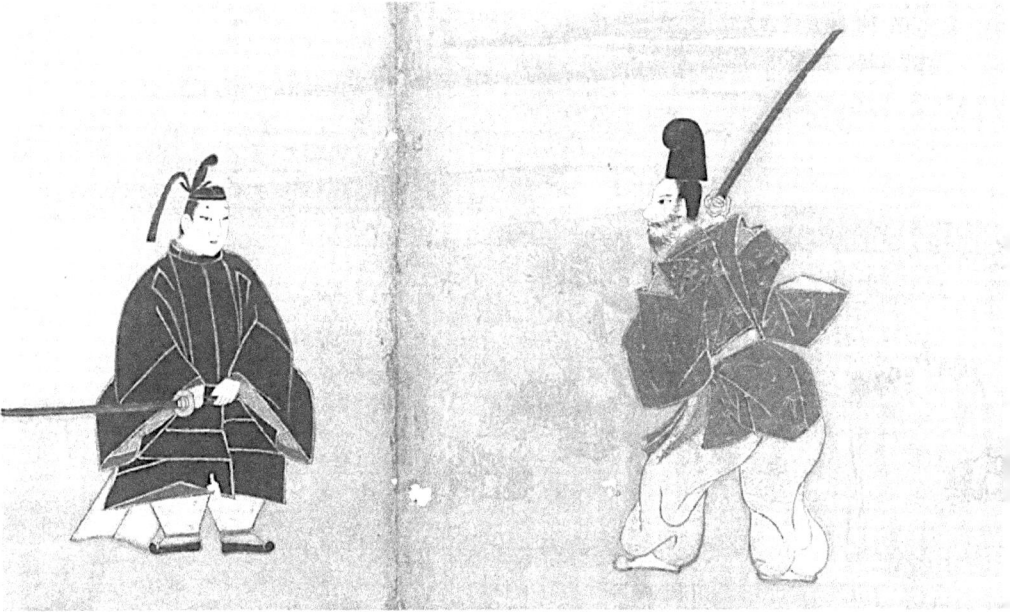

Jigen Ryu Scroll
Edo Era

Haebaru Ueekata of Onaka Town (Nowadays the Yokoda Household) was a martial arts master and the man who introduced Jigen School sword to Okinawa.[16]

One day Morishima Ueekata [17] (the father of Giwan Choho) and Morishima's student, Haneji Aji went to watch Haebaru's training. Morishima commented in a cool, authoritative way,

This does not seem particularly effective.

Word of this comment reached Haebaru Sensei and, having been insulted to his face, immediately challenged Morishima to a duel to the death.

Thus, it came to pass that both men presented themselves in the main room of Oroku Udon's residence, wearing court dress.[18] Both men were handed Shinken, live blades, and apparently all the women were beside themselves.

Morishima Ueekata immediately apologized for his brazen insult and that same day he, along with his friend Haneji Aji, both joined Hebaru Ueekata's Dojo and began training.

As you can see, people long ago, were very serious about responding to insults to their art. Innumerable famous Samurai have recorded such episodes their memoirs, which are still appearing today.

---

[16] Haebaru Ueekata 南風原親方守周 A retainer of the Shimazu Clan in Kyushu in the late 17th ~ early 18th century.

[17] Giwan Choho 宜湾 朝保 （1823~1876）

[18] Oroku Udon 小禄御殿 a royal lineage descended from Urasoe Choman 浦添朝満 （1494~1540） the eldest son of King Shino 尚真 王(1465~1527.) The family traditionally served as Daimyo, regional governors.

に依れば大中の南風原親方（今の真古田の屋敷）は示現流の鼻祖で武術の達人であつたさうた所が或日のこと森島義方（宜湾朝保の父）其門人羽地按司の修練するのを見て限……ものを知つた……何の役に立つかと冷かされた其音が先生の耳に入り法を誘るなら自分が目前に於て決闘するに如かやと先生大禮服を着けられ小藏御殿のお廣間に於て両人に異剣を渡し女性衆方をさわがしたさうだそまで森島親方は其過音を詫まり即日より羽地按司のお中間……て共に南風原親方に付て稽古をされたさうである者の人……はれ程法を重せられたの……た記憶のまゝに記して見れば赤田の奥田山川の松元（今の大鉢嶺の屋敷）佐渡山親方同じアザーダンメー弟の目小松村親雲上、弟松村營藏の大村赤平の石嶺、儀保の石嶺、金城、徳嶺今歸八仁小、金城の大田、外間親雲上、豊見

娘親方、久塲川の大城、親泊、仲宗根浦崎、鳥小堀の鉄拳金城、多和田、大中ハ漢那、豊見山眞和志の上原口小、汀志良次の尾嘉比小添石、泉崎の崎山（汀志良次眞玉橋の官生供）其志親雲上（豊見鳩親方の師匠）上里、阿波連、宮里小、東の右術門殿の鳩袋、九年母屋の比嘉、桑江小、西ぃ長濱、久米の湖城小、前里、泊の城間、金城、山里、仲里、伊波、親泊、松茂良、前川、山田、知念志喜屋仲、津堅ハンタ小、古波藏宮平、佐敷の屋比久主（地頭）等ハ何れも皆知名の武術家で尚敬王と尚瀨王は器主キの勇君であられた鉄拳宮城は尚敬王の御附武官で松村親雲上は尚瀨王の侍徒武官

一日尚濱王は古謝按司（今の美里按司の祖父）に如何です今日私のカメジア（松村の童名を愛して云はれたお名葉）と合手になれるものが居るかとお〻間になつたさところが古謝按司は早速松村と私等はあまり甲乙はありませんか大義を得たる者

The following are all famous martial artists: [19]

赤田の奥田	Okuta of Akata
山川の松元	Matsumoto of Yamakawa (Currently in a house in Ohachimine)
佐渡山親方	Sadoyama Ueekata is also in Ohachimine
アザータンメー弟の目小	
	Megusuku, Brother of Azaatanmee
松村親雲上	Matsumura Pechin
弟松村当蔵の大村	
	His brother Matsumura Tonoku of Omura
赤平の石嶺	Ishimine of Akahira
儀保の石嶺	Ishimine of Giho
金城	Kinjo
徳嶺今帰仁小	Tokumine Nakijin
久場川の大城	Kubakawa no Ogusuku
親泊	Oyatomari
仲宗根浦崎	Nakasone Urazaki
島子堀の鉄拳金城	Shimakobori no Tekken Kinjo
多和田	Tawada
大中	Onaka
漢那	Kanna
豊見山真和志の上原口小 （汀志良次真玉橋の官生供）	
	Toyomiyama Mawashi no Ueharaguchi Sho (Terashiraji Hashi Kansho)
具志親雲上 (豊見城親方の師匠)	
	Kushi Pechin (The teacher of Toyomi Gusuku Ueekata)
上里	Kamizato
阿波連	Aharen

---

[19] There are no readings given to these names, they are the most likely reading based on the translator's research.

官里小	Kanzato Sho
東右衛門殿の島袋	Higashi Uemon Dono no Shimabukuro
九年母屋の比嘉	Kunenboya of Higa
桑江小	Kuwae Sho
西の長濱	Nagahama of Nishi
久米の湖城小	Kogusuku Sho of Kume
前里	Maezato
泊の城間	Gusukuma of Tomari
金城	Kinjo
山里	Yamazato
仲里	Nakazato
伊波	Inami
親泊	Oyatomari
松茂良	Matsumora
前田	Maeda
山田	Yamata
知念志喜屋仲	Chinenshikiyanaka
津堅ハンタ小	Tsuken Hantasho
古波蔵宮平	Kohagura Miyahira
佐敷の屋比久主(地頭)	Yabikuni no Shu of Sashiki (Head of Region)

King Shokei and King Shoko[20] both chose brave warriors from amongst their regional Daimyo.

---

[20] King Shokei   尚敬王 (1700 ~ 1751)

King Shoko   尚灝王 (1787 ~ 1834)

古謝按司（今の美里按司の祖父）に如何
ですか今日私のカメジア（松村の童名を
愛して云はれたお言葉）と合手になれ
るものが居るかとお尋ねになつたあと
がある古謝按司は早速松村と私等はあ
まり甲乙はありませんか大義を得た者
が勝ちでありますと恭しく答へられた
尚瀬王は流石は武士であると大うろ
譽めになつたあとかあられたさうです
其外摩文仁按司小禄按司等を貴族方て
の武士て現在生存しとる中では糸洲親
雲上（師範中學の唐手教師）西い東恩納
小（水産、商校の唐手教師）裏の東恩納
泊の安謝間の嶋袋、久茂地の新垣小
湧田の安謝間の嶋袋・久茂地の新垣小
桃原の東風平親方、島小堀の桑江、金
城の山口（御新筆今は垣花）山根の知念
（現住垣花）屋部（師範校武術教師）花城
（一中校武術教師）等であらう屋部花城
の如く教育的に系統だつて唐手を研究
名を轟かすであらう（松濤）

Tekken "Iron Fist" Miyagi served as the *O-Fubukan*, aide-de-camp to King Shokei. [21] Matsumura Pechin[22] served as *Jiju Bukan* aide-de-camp to King Shoko.

One day King Shokei commented to the Kosha Anji, the administrator of the Kosha area,

Do you know anyone who can cross hands with Kamejia?

(Kamejia is the name Matsumura had as a child, which the King used as a friendly nickname.)[23]

The administrator replied immediately,

As far as skill goes, it is hard to say if Matsumura's art is better than ours, however surely the person with greater moral authority will emerge victorious.

King Shokei was impressed at this polite response and commented,

An answer worthy of a warrior!

---

[21] *O-Fubukan* 御付武官 aide-de-camp to the King. Also known as a Jiju Bukan 侍従武官 whose primary duties are to report military affairs to the Emperor and act as a close attendant. In the Ryukyu Kingdom he also taught martial arts to the royal family.

[22] Matsumura Sokon 松村宗棍 (1809? ~ 1899?)

[23] Brackets are by Funakoshi Gichin.

In addition, there are other members of the royal family like Mabuni Aji, Shoroku Aji and so on. Among the currently active marital artists there is Itosu Pechin (Currently a Karate instructor at the Junior High Instructor's School) Nishi no Higashionna (Currently a Karate Instructor at a Fishing and Commerce School)[24] and Higashi no Higashionna. [25]

Shimabukuro of Kuwata Ajama, of Aragaki of Kumoji, Yamada of Anri Kodomari, Toyomiyama of Onaka, Kochinda Ueekata of Tobaru, Kuwae of Tonju, Yamaguchi of Kinjo (Formerly the scribe-secretary[26] to the king, currently Kakihana.) Chinen of Yamane (Nowadays known as Kakihana,) Yabu (a martial arts instructor at the teacher's college)[27] Hanagusuku (a martial arts instructor at First Junior High School)[28] and others.

In particular, instructors like Yabu and Hanagusuku organize their Karate training from an educational standpoint.

By Shoto.

---

[24] Higaonna Kanryo   東恩納寛量 (1853 ~ 1915) Known as West Higashionna.

[25] Higaonna Kanryu (1849 ~1922) Known as East Higashionna.

[26] *Goyuhitsu* 御祐筆 official scribe-secretary. Person charged with writing official letters, poems and recording the King's diary. Also refers to the Oku Goyuhitsu, who does the same for the wife of the king.

[27] Yabu Kentsu   屋部憲通 (1866 ~ 1937)

[28] Hanagusuku Chomo 花城長茂 (1869 ~ 1945)

Okinawa no Bugi
The Martial Arts of Okinawa
Regarding Karate: Regarding What Asato Anko Told Me
By Shoto
Ryukyu Shinpo Newspaper
January 18th 1914

(Part 2 of 3)
Karate no Ryugi
The Different Schools of Karate

●沖繩の武技（中）

唐手に就いて、　安里安恒氏談

▲唐手の流儀には昭霊流と照林流の二通りあるが前は体軀肥満にして体力豊富なる偉大の男がやるべきものにして「アツン」（武官）はあれに屬し後は体力貧弱にして術に置きを置く痩方の男が多くやるべきものにして「ツイシンザン」（武官）はあの流儀であつた現今我が沖縄で中等學校の生徒等がやるのを見ると那覇、稽古したのは多く昭林流で首里で稽古したのは多く照林流

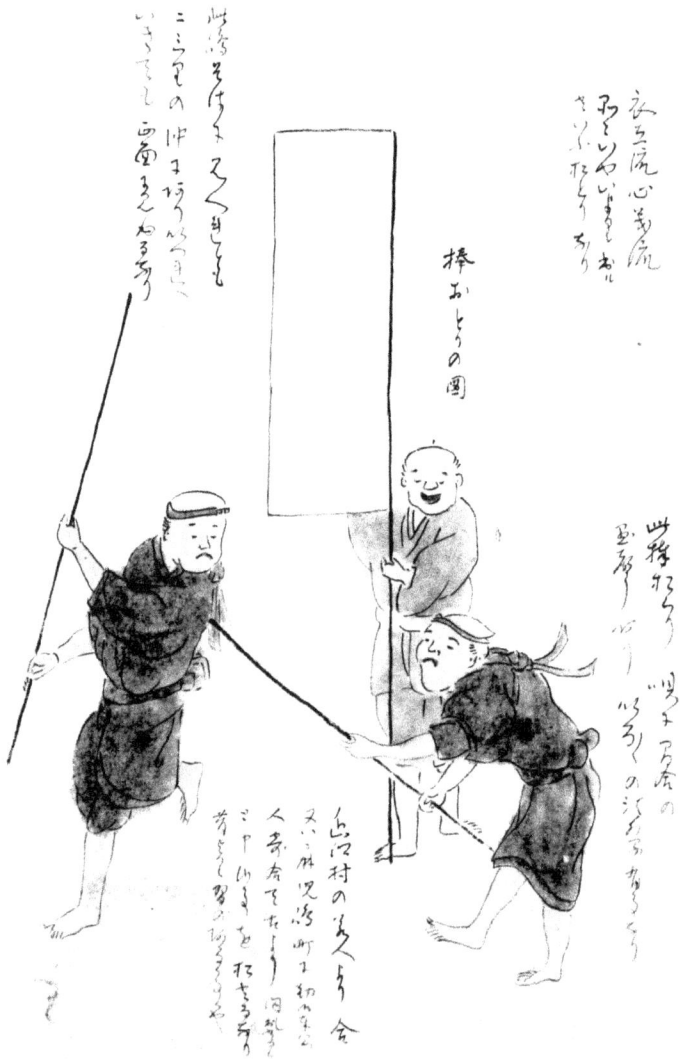

*The wooden staff dance is popular. It is done by singing and beating
the poles in unison. Samurai and townsfolk alike have danced
together in Kagoshima from long ago.*

Satsuma Fudoki 薩摩風土記 Record of Satsuma Traditions.

(Part 2 of 3)
Karate no Ryugi
The Different Schools of Karate

There are two schools Shorei Ryu and Shorin Ryu. The former is best done by large men who are blessed with strength and have fat bodies. Ason (a Bukan, Chinese military commander) is associated with that style of Karate. The latter is an art mostly done by those who are thin and weak. Waishinzan (a Bukan, Chinese military commander) is associated with that style of Karate.

Currently in Okinawan junior high schools in the Naha region, most do Shorei Ryu Karate while in Shuri the training is mostly in Shorin Ryu. The reason is the focus of each area is different. In Naha they place a greater importance on physical power while in Shuri they are more partial to technical skill. This is simply a difference in approach, and one way is not bad while the other is good.

It is it is important to correctly evaluate the physical condition and body type of the learner and adjust your lesson accordingly. If you do not carefully choose the proper learning materials and style of lesson, it will end up making teaching difficult and progress will be slow. Further, it could well cause injury to the learner.

Regarding the techniques in Karate, if you counted them all up, there are dozens of different ones. However, it is not necessary to memorize each and every one of them. Further, it is not necessary to memorize many techniques. It is enough to select five or six techniques and train them thoroughly. If you wish to strengthen and firm your body then techniques like Naifanchi and Seesan are best. If you want to defend against Bo, wooden staff, then Passai is the only option available. If you want to work on reaction time, then Kunsangun is best.

The technique Jitte teaches how to differentiate and defend against upper, middle and lower attacks. However, as far as what the most applicable in real life techniques are, I would say Seesan and the Tomari version of Passai are extremely effective.

The completely the wrong approach to Karate is thinking that spending a great deal of time learning many techniques is an indication of proficiency.

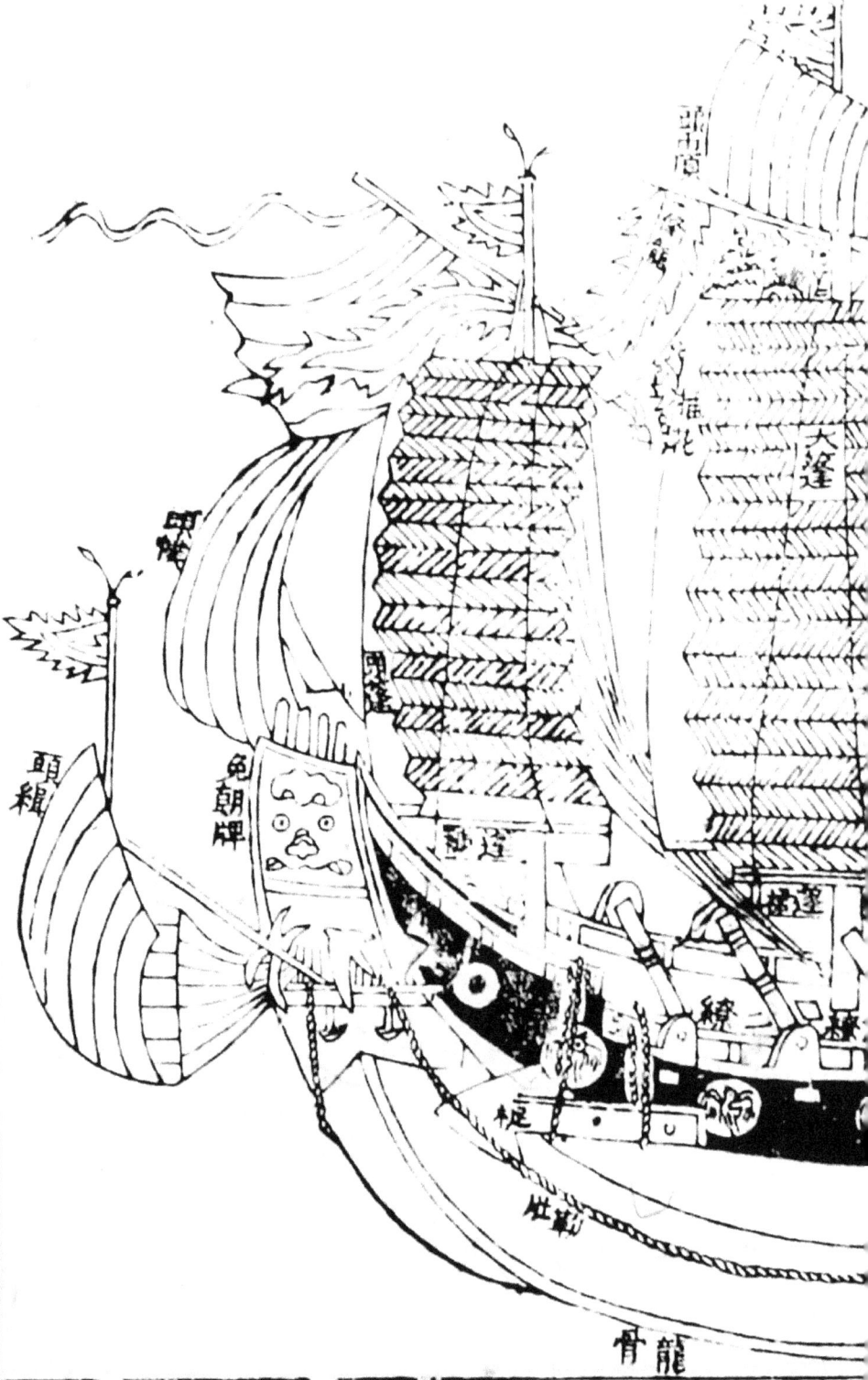

圖繪

頭緝

頭巾

龜朗牌

船篷

大篷

碇

舵

壮舡

龍骨

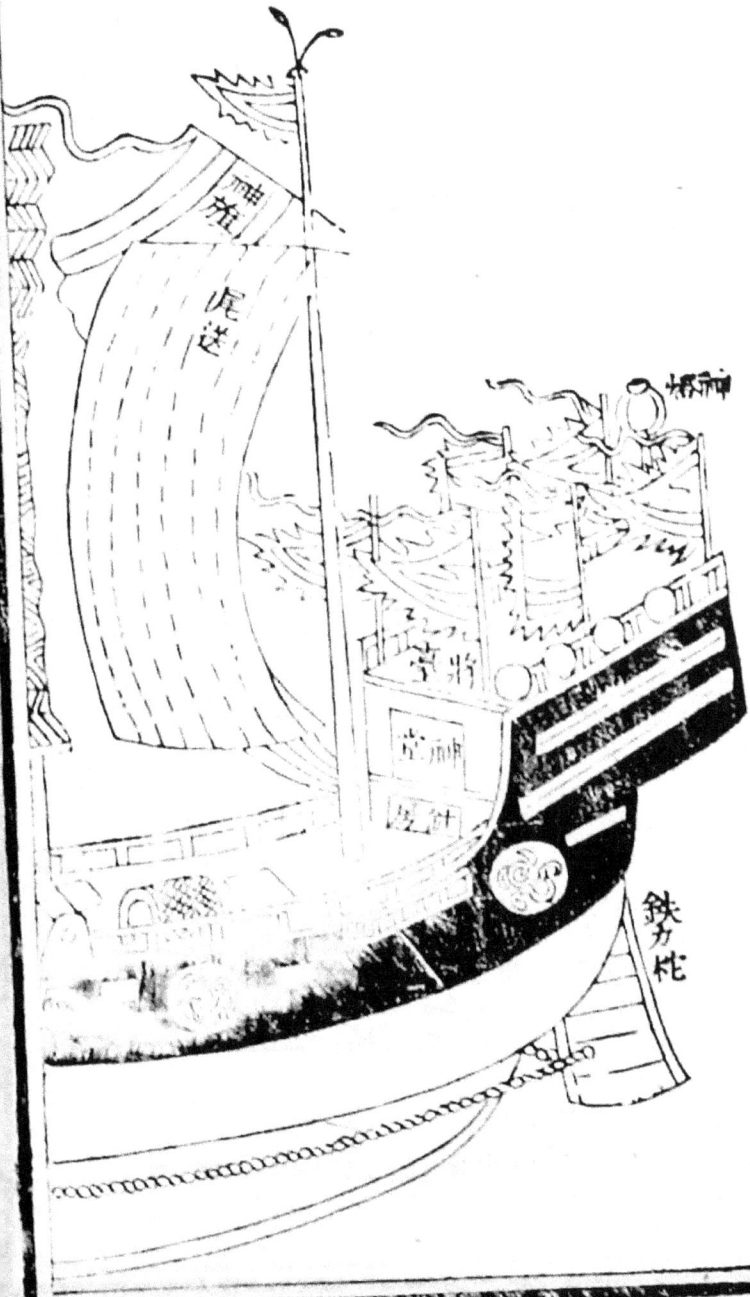

▲唐手の種類　数へ擧ぐれは数十種もあるが悉く覺えらるゝものではないぶ亦さう澤山覺ゆる必要もないのだ其中上五六種撰擇してよく練習しさへすれはそれで充分だ休を固める向には「ナイハンチ」と「セーサン」が好からう棒を受けるものは「バッサイ」に限るナ早き上段中段下段の區別を判然したのは「セ

「ジッテ」である而して實用向には「ク…ンサンクン」が徐程利くやうにあるなかなかちりをして徐く知つてゐると得意がるのは甚た

▲直接傳授を受けた人　支那に往き或は本縣にて直接支那人より傳授を受けた人が多數あるが「アソン」の弟子には泉崎の﨑山（豐見城親方の師匠）長濱友寄具志親雲上（儀保の石嶺の師匠）「イワー」の弟子には首里の松村親雲上久米の米・前里湖城小「ワイシンザン」の弟子には東の右衛門殿の島袋九年毋屋の比嘉・今の比嘉德の父）西の東恩納小深等

した﨑州安南の人より稽古したのが府の城間と金城は「チント―」山里は「ヂーシ」仲里は「チンテ―」山里は「チント―」松村と親泊は

People Who Received Direct Transmission[29]

There are a great number of people who either went to China and received direct instruction or received instruction from a Chinese person in our prefecture. Students of Ason are Sakiyama of Izumizaki (teacher of Tomigusuku Ueekata,) Nagahama Tomoyose Gushichin Pechin (the teacher of Ishimine of Giho.)

The students of Iwaa were Matsumura Pechin of Shuri and Kume of Maeri and Kogusuku Sho.[30]

The students of Waishinzan were Shimabukuro of Higashi Uemondono and Higa of Kunenboya (The father of Higatoku, who is around today) and Nishi Higashionna.

The man from An'nan region of Fuzhou, China whose ship drifted into Tomari port was in a hurry to return home to China and thus taught different techniques to different people.

---

[29] Illustration on the previous pages shows the type of Ryukyu Ship that transported tribute to Imperial China. Due to the system at the time, Ryukyu received goods in return from Imperial that exceeded the value of their tribute. From the *Ryukyu kokushi ryaku* 琉球国志略 an abbreviated history of the Ryukyu Kingdom. Edo Era.

[30] Maeri of Kume is probably Shinezato Ranbo 眞栄里蘭芳 (1838-1904) There are many Kogusuku 湖城 in this era, so it is hard to say who this is, possibly Kogusuku Shuren 湖城秀連氏 (1883~1945.)

The techniques were divided up as follows:

- Gusukuma of Tomari as well as Kanagusuku were taught Chinto.[31]
- Matsumura and Oyadomari were taught Chinti.[32]
- Yamazato was taught Jiin[33] and Nakazato was taught Jitte.

The reason the area around the port of Tomari has comparatively more families who specialize in martial arts dates to the feudal era. As the port was only a couple of miles from Shuri, families in that area were officially allowed to practice martial arts by the Shuri Government, so they could be called upon should there be a sudden attack.

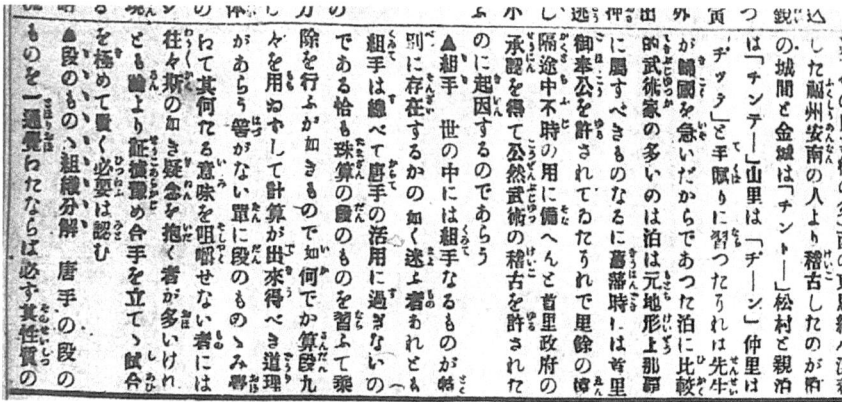

Kumite
Paired Training

Kumite, paired training, holds a particular place in the martial arts world. For those not familiar with the word "Kumite," it is nothing more than the systematic application of Karate techniques. Just like when you learn to calculate figures on an abacus or do multiplication. Clearly you are not going to be able to understand the fundamental

---

[31] Chinto is written as Chintoo チントー

[32] This may be a misprint, not Matsumura but Matsumora Kosaku 松茂良興作(1829~1898) and Kokan Oyadomari 親泊興寛 (1827 ~ 1905) Chinti is recorded as Chintee チンテー

[33] Jiin ジーン

principles of mathematics if you don't first learn the 9 x 9 multiplication tables. Thus, Kumite is simply to be memorized at one stage on the path of learning.

There can be many who do not comprehend this or have various doubts and questions; however, evidence is better than theory, thus such people should cross hands with an opponent in a Shiai, duel.

Levels in Karate and an Explanation of the Organization

If you learn how each stage of learning in Karate works, you will invariably develop an understanding of its essence of how the organization is arranged. So, in answer to the questions, "What is this part of?" "What is that part of?" The first thing to understanding this is keep that curious mindset while training.

When you first start training, you should not put any power into your strikes and instead focus on memorizing the body movements. Once you have learned the mechanics of a technique, practice putting seventy percent of your power into each strike, thereby expanding your understanding. Putting in power from the very beginning is premature, as your will not be able to fully absorb the lesson.

Eventually, once you have achieved greater proficiency, you should sometimes train with just twenty percent of your power. Other times train with only fifty percent of your power.

When demonstrating your technique in front of people, I believe it is ideal to use about seventy percent of your power.

By Shoto

Okinawa no Bugi
The Martial Arts of Okinawa
Regarding Karate: Regarding What Asato Anko Told Me
By Shoto

Ryukyu Shinpo Newspaper
January 19th 1914

(Part 3 of 3)
Renshuchu no Kokoroe
Things To Consider When Training

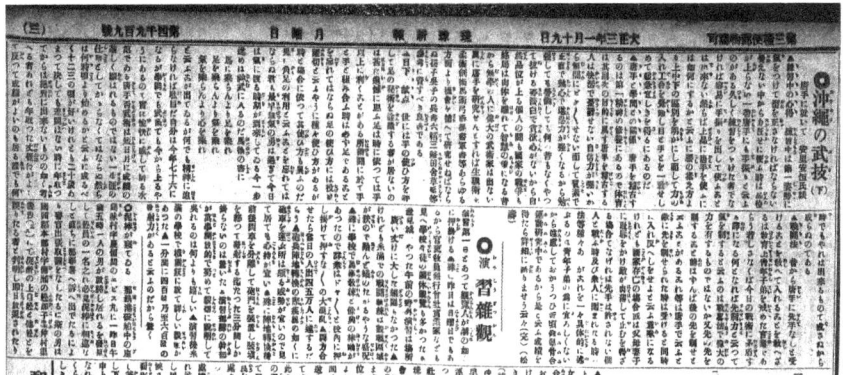

Okinawa no Bugi
The Martial Arts of Okinawa
Regarding Karate: Regarding What Asato Anko Told Me
By Shoto

(Part 3 of 3)
Renshuchu no Kokoroe
Things To Consider When Training

The most important thing to focus on while training is your posture as without it you can't do Kata properly. You will never develop refined Karate if you put power in the technique before you actually have the technique itself memorized.

For example, you must train a given set of hand and arm movements extensively, failing to do this means you won't be able to easily employ that technique.

So, then what must you do in order to achieve refined Karate? The answer is being able to correctly position your hips in either upper, middle or lower position, depending on the technique as well as being aware of how and when to apply power. By combining proper hip placement while your eyes and hands operate in unison, you will be able to execute techniques at the proper tempo, slow or fast, depending on the situation.[34]

The Relationship Between Karate and Scholarship

The most important thing in martial arts is developing a strong focused mind, while physical fitness is the second objective. People that train Karate do not suffer from depression and, as they have a powerful self-confidence, they do not react impulsively. As Karate practitioners are reserved, direct and passionate people with a powerful endurance, they are able to complete any task set before them, whether it is work or study, without any undue strain.

---

[34] *Kan-Kyu* 緩急 fast and slow. Applies to all martial arts as well as performance arts. Often mentioned in conjunction with *Kyo-Jaku* 強弱 strength and weakness, power and softness.

大砲鍛錬図

川崎家の大砲南蛮傳
位して其後南蛮祖父傳を
継て今に島人ども鍛練す
る事なり

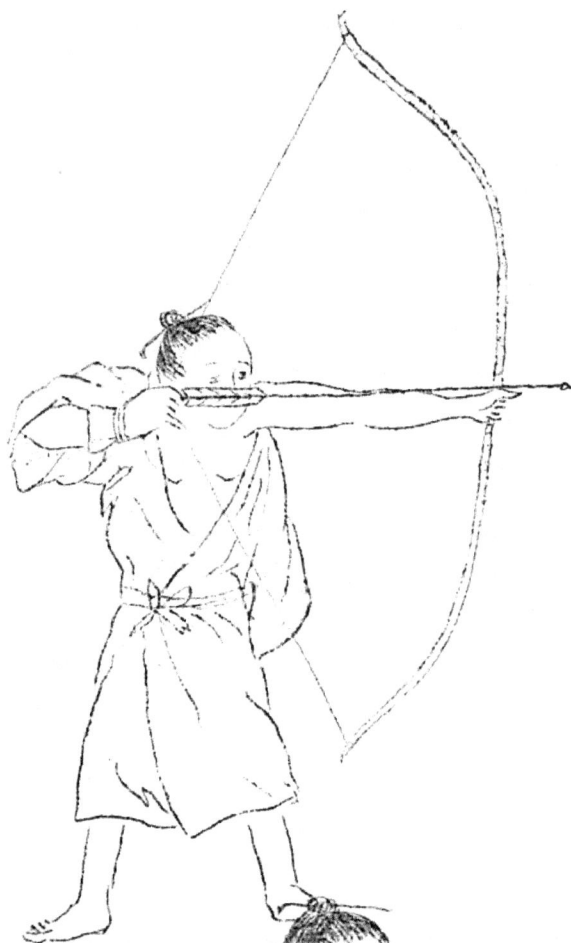

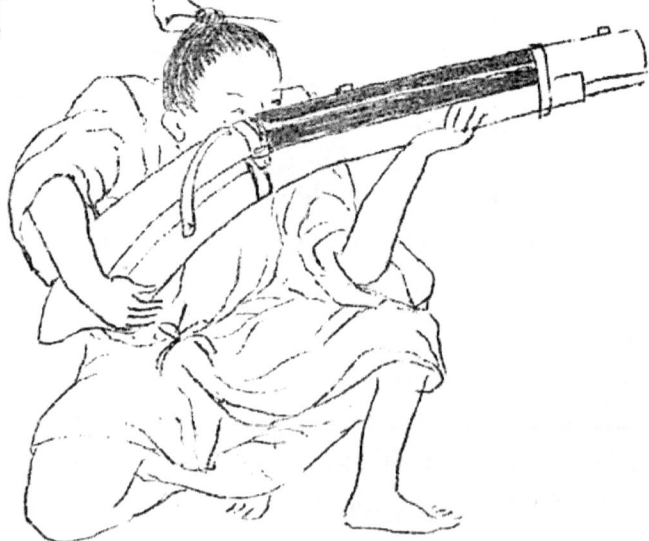

As the character of Karate practitioners is straightforward and without greed, they naturally develop into more refined people. Further, they do not engage in personal fights or battles between nations. In the end, they do not rely on physical combat, but rather a battle of intellect.

Long ago, uneducated men could never rise to lead a great martial arts family. If you are serious about training Karate then, to fully develop yourself, it is necessary to learn Jujutsu, Kenjutsu, Bajutsu, Kyujutsu along with reading military and strategy books.[35] In short, you must take every chance to learn things from every subject. This includes reading Sun Tzu's *Art of War*, Wu Qi's *The Wuzi* as well as *The Six Secret Teachings and The Three Strategies* of Huang Shigong [36] in addition to books like *A Scroll Regarding the Countryside*.[37] All of these are excellent resources and good books to keep on hand.[38]

Areas That Are Lacking[39]

The fact that there are many experts who will comment on how to use the hands, but none that delve into the inner mysteries of utilizing the legs is extremely unfortunate. There are times when using your feet is much more effective than using your hands.

When you are in a duel, and trading blows with your opponent, forget to use your feet at your own peril.

---

[35] Jujutsu, Sword Fighting, Equestrian Arts, Archery.

[36] *The Art of War, The Wuzi* and *The Six Secret Teachings* are all part of The Seven Military Classics.

[37] Illustration on following pages showing a naked tattooed woman running amok from Inaka Zoshi 田舎草紙 *A Scroll Regarding the Countryside* is a comical story published in 1809 by Juppensha Ikku 十返舎一九 (1765~1831.)

[38] Illustration on previous page:
Nanto Zatsuwa 南島雑話 Tales From the Southern Isles 1855
Illustration showing matchlock and archery training in Oshima. The matchlock school was introduced by the Kawasaki Family.

[39] There is a Kanji missing in the original, so the meaning is not entirely clear.

大もり

女のしやう
ても色ん
きのつを
りすくく
まこつくるま
ひますわした

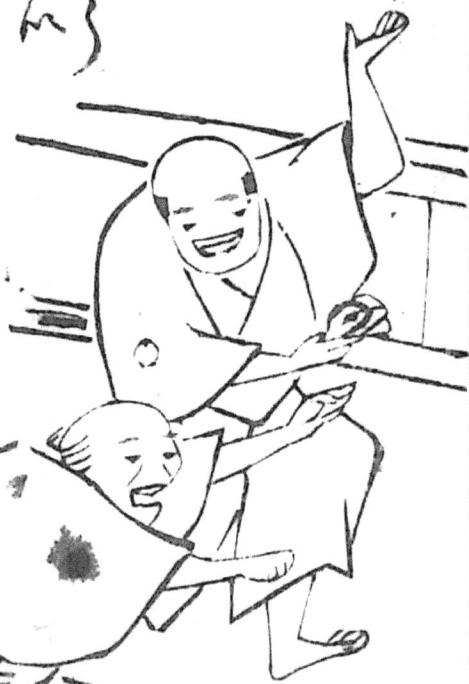
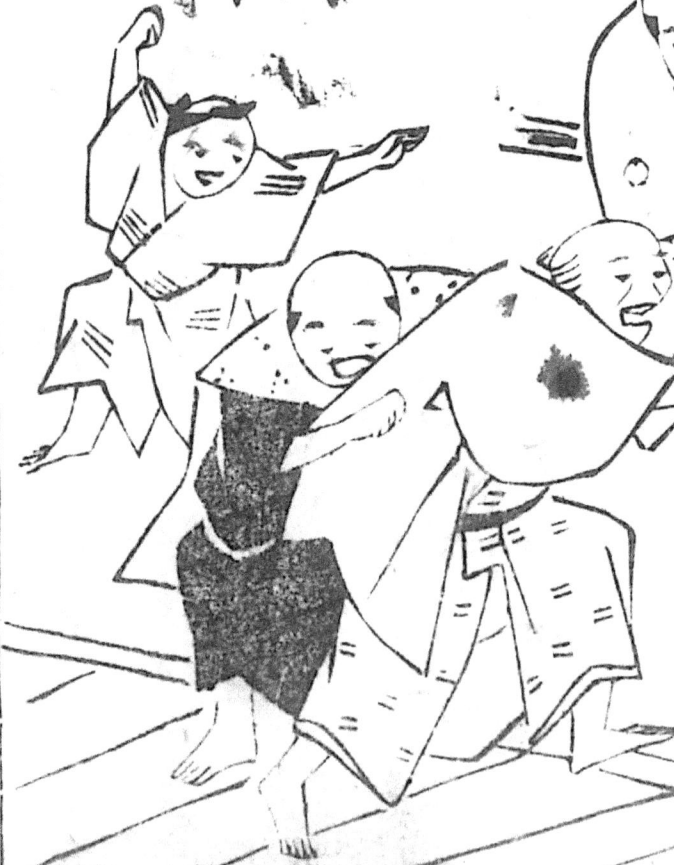

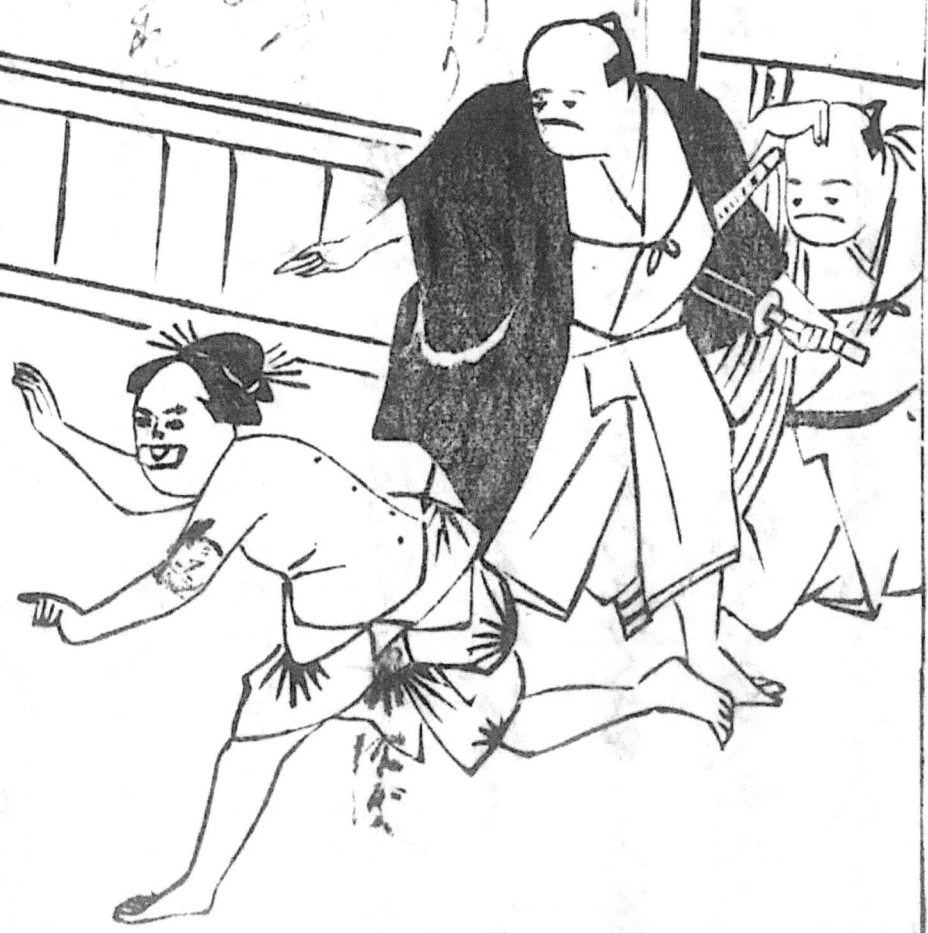

There are all sorts of ways to use your feet like Nage Ashi or Fumi Kiri, Leap In, however the method you select and the way you apply it depends on the situation. In short, you must not forget to employ your feet.

You have lost much of the vigor of youth and now you are in a calmer state of mind and are only one step away from achieving a nearly divine level of cultured martial ability. There is a certain Bajutsu, equestrian art, scroll that states,

Instead of riding a horse, travel upon your legs
Instead of travelling on your legs, use the wave of your martial energy
Instead of using the wave of your martial enemy, ride your mind

You cannot allow everything to overwhelm you and drain your focus. This year I turn seventy-six years old, despite that I feel I am easily progressing not only in my martial arts but also in academic study. In Karate, and all martial arts really, progress cannot be made in just a few days or months, rather it is the work of an entire lifetime.

As for when the best time would be to start Karate, I would say that around twelve or thirteen years of age would be ideal, however starting at twenty poses no problem. As far as "at what age would it be impossible to start" I would have to say as long as you know your limits, anyone can start at any time.

How to Fight

From days long past it has been taught that Karate doesn't make the first strike, and only blocks. This is done as part of the educational curriculum in order to serve as a warning to the young students. That being said it is a bit inconsistent with regards to the arts of war. For example, clearly there is an advantage to making the first strike in order to take control of a duel and this can apply to strategically pressuring your opponent in order gain a significant advantage in a battle.

If using Sen no Sen, correctly identifying your opponent's method of attack and moving to attack before he can launch his strike, does not work then you should employ Go no Sen, waiting for your opponent to attack before launching your own strike. In Karate, when an opponent overcomes you with Sen no Sen, you simply block and respond with your attack in the exact same instant.

Unless someone is threatening the very existence of the country or some villain is threatening to bring shame upon your parents, wife or children, or perhaps you suddenly find yourself in a close quarter combat situation and have no choice, then you cannot strike first.

In fact, the law varies regarding individuals fighting, or when people are surrounded by a mob. Explaining to youths the ins and outs of the law for each and every one of these situations is not going to be helpful, so a simple rule is used instead.

I am currently doing research related to exercises that work the respiratory system and will be reporting on it in detail.

End

By Shoto

Ryukyu Kenpo Karate
Funakoshi Gichin
Public Physical Education Resources
市民体育資料 1924

八、琉球拳法唐手

富 名 腰 義 珍

平和克復の今日でも、運動體育は最も必要なので、益々隆盛を極むるやうな傾向がある。けれども、其種に依り選擇を誤るときは、或は圓滿なる心身の發達を缺ぐの嫌ひあるので、余は茲に其缺陷を補はんが爲めに全身均齊に發達する體育運動法たると共に、又最も安全にして簡易なる護身術として、我が琉球拳法「唐手」を軍隊、學校、青年團、及び一般家庭運動法として提供する譯である。

組織 その主目的を別ちて體育、護身、精神修養の三とす。(一)體育としての「唐手」術は眼、

Ryukyu Kenpo Karate
Funakoshi Gichin
1924

Even though we have gone to great effort to bring about peace, physical education is still of paramount importance and, indeed, the trend towards greater fitness is continuing to flourish. However, people may choose the wrong method and end up training in a way that does not develop their body and mind in a comprehensive and unified manner, which leads to dissatisfaction.

I would like to introduce the Ryukyu Kenpo physical fitness system which evenly develops all parts of the body, without any deficiencies. It is called "Karate" and it is also a method of self-defense which is the safest and simplest you can learn. I am offering this system to the military, schools, youth groups as well as to everyday folks to use as a method of exercise to do at home.

Organization

Karate is divided into three primary objectives: Physical Education, Self-Defense and Developing Fighting Spirit.

Physical Education

All parts of the body are exercised evenly when training Karate. This includes the eyes, neck, chest, upper body, lower body. Proper breathing and jumping are also taught. When training you will stretch all parts of the body, meaning the very core of body will become more flexible. You will learn how to shift your body to any point you choose, by either advancing, moving sideways or moving diagonally. This is a method of exercise that teaches how to accurately employ speed and power. Truly, this is a standardized, systematic art that is quite fascinating.

Though there are many styles of exercise that are popular now, they often focus on one aspect to excess, meaning there is a danger some element is lacking and your conditioning won't be comprehensive. Not only can Karate succeed in developing your body evenly, but it is also the most comprehensive and healthy methodology.

A Collection of Karatedo 空手道集成
Keio University Karate Club 慶応義塾体育会空手部
1936

Te Gatana – Hand Sword	Hirakubi/Heito – Base of Palm
裏刀 手刀	平頭 （三十七）
Enpi – Monkey Elbow	**Left: Seiken – True Fist** **Right: Waki Ken – Side Fist**
猿臂 （三十九）	正拳 脇拳

Self-Defense

Practicing the above-mentioned exercises will enable you to use Karate as a method of self-defense. When faced with an unavoidable situation you can use Yubi-Gatana (finger strike,) Kenkotsu (fist,) Hirakubi/Heito (palm) Enpi (elbow) and feet to defend yourself as appropriate. Not only can Karate be used in place of a weapon to defend yourself, but you can also use this method to protect others. In short it is a martial art you can easily employ if a situation arises.

Developing the Spirit

The morality taught in Karate is in line with what is taught to all Japanese citizen, namely, the same commitment to loyalty and filial piety that forms the basis for the Bushido spirit. Karate reveres bravery, prioritizes being true to your principles, having proper manners, offering proper respect, being loyal, faithful and consistent. Further, the Karate training develops unparalleled bravery and the ability to endure hardship while remaining honorable, charitable, diligent, tenacious and persistent.

Clearly Karate is a system that is completely in line with the founding principles of the nation of Japan and thus is inseparable from the spirit of the Japanese people. Considering that, of late, there are many people in society who act rashly and with almost no consideration of their actions, we sorely need to direct people's interest towards absorbing this method of old-style martial arts. Thus, no matter how you look at the situation, Karate is not something that *should* be done, but is something that is *essential*.

Age

Whether you are a boy or a girl, if you begin training from around ten to sixteen years of age, it won't harm your physical development in any way. That being said, hard Karate training can probably only be endured by those from around fifteen to people in their forties. Further, conducting training appropriate to your body throughout your life will not result in any ill effects and will, in fact, likely act as preventative medicine.

Place

The time you need to spend training is very short. To learn the first technique the average person will only need about two hours. If you are particularly adept at learning, you'll be able to get a firm grasp of a Kata in less than an hour. Typically, when conducting training you only need two minutes to perform each Kata, thus no matter how busy you may be, if you have a commitment to training, you can take time in the morning, evening or even during break times.

Conclusion

Karate Can be done by men women old and young, either by yourself or as part of a group. It can be done in any place, doesn't require any money, is not dangerous, develops your physical body, provides you with a form of self-defense and develops mental fortitude. As the mysterious saying goes, *the weak become powerful and life is extended and preserved for eternity.*

Additional Material

History

Throughout the history of our Ryukyu islands, martial arts were banned twice. The first was long ago when King Sho Shin (1465 ~ 1527) consolidated power in Shuri. At that time, he ordered that all weapons be turned in, thereby reducing the power of the regional lords. The second time was following the Keicho Campaign of 1609, when Ryukyu became a vassal of Satsuma Domain and the lord of Satsuma Domain banned the sale of weapons. This meant that, following the invasion, the Ryukyu people had few opportunities to train martial arts. The intent of this policy was to keep the population peaceful and docile.

The natural result of these historical pressures was that the people began to study how to protect themselves against enemies despite being unarmed. In other words, Karate is *Mutekatsu Ryu Ryukyu Kenpo*, Fighting Style of the Ryukyu Islands: Victory While Unarmed School.

Origin

According to academic Koda Rohan,[40]

> *Ken no Ho*, The Way of the Fist, is part of the Shorin religious practice. Shorinji Temple is where Zen sprouted and later it became the source from which the Kenpo method spread. Following the beginning of the Ming era (1368~1644) there were many novels and collections of writings that discussed the incomparable strength of Shorinji fighting. Things such as a Shorinji practitioner being able to strike with one finger and kill a person. Or that a single strike with a closed fist can knock a man down. Xie Zhaozhe[41] wrote, "The Kenpo of Shorinji Temple is unparalleled under the heavens. Monks from that temple travelled out in every direction and each of them could best dozens of men."

By reading these excerpts it becomes clear that Kenpo originated long in the past at Shorinji Temple and that Kenpo itself emerged from Zen practices. Thus, believing that Kenpo only came to Ryukyu following the Keicho Invasion by Satsuma in 1609 seems doubtful.

Schools of Karate

The schools of Karate can be divided into two broad categories: Shorin Ryu and Shorei Ryu. It seems likely that Shorin Ryu is an abbreviation of Shorinji Temple Style and Shorei Ryu is an abbreviation of Shoreiji Temple Style. The name of the latter seems to describe a fighting technique "that has been drawn into the body and unified with spirit." In later generations, schools took the name of masters of the art and a great many sub-schools diverged from there. However, all schools are related to the two original styles. Each has its own unique characteristics and if you employ the best part of each for a good purpose and unify your body and mind you will easily reach

---

[40] Koda Rohan 幸田露伴 is the pen name of Koda Shigeyuki 幸田成行 (1867 ~ 1947)

[41] Xie Zhaozhe 謝肇淛 (1567~1624)

a state where you will be able to respond to any attack by moving freely and uninhibited in any direction.

Value

Long ago Karate was a closely guarded secret, however starting in the 34th or 35th year of Meiji, 1901~1902, an interesting thing happened. When doctors were giving physical fitness evaluations to students, as well as new recruits for the army, they were startled by what they found. Both the students and the young military recruits had extremely well-developed bodies. The officer in charge reported this to the Department of Education. With that, Karate became an official part of the physical education program at schools. Now that energy has spread rapidly throughout the country.

One example of this startling development is a schoolteacher who took his students' measurements after three months of training. He found, on average, that their torso had increased in size by 1 Sun, an inch, and their body weight had increased by 600 Monme, a pound. While this is but a single example, there are many community Karate groups as well as school groups. Once school begins, I plan on having the school doctor measure the students and then several months later measure them again and compare the results. My eventual goal is to collate this data and release it to the public.

Honors

Mr. Hojo Jiju was able to speak to His Majesty the Emperor regarding Karate, and, thanks to his good offices, on March 6th of Taisho 10 (1921) when the crown prince[42] travelled to Okinawa prefecture we were blessed with the honor of his presence at our demonstration which he commented positively on.[43]

I heard that last year (1923) when the crown prince Hirohito visited Taiwan, he inquired of the administrator whether there was a martial art native to Taiwan like Karate is native to Ryukyu. In conclusion, we have been blessed that our Ryukyu Kenpo Karate has been seen by both the Taisho Emperor and Empress, further it was our great honor to have Crown Prince Hirohito view one of our demonstrations. Truly we are showered with blessings.

Critique

The late Marquise Sho Tai, the last King of the Ryukyu Kingdom, was known as "a man of robust health." The eighth Tokugawa Shogun Tokugawa Yoshimune was known for promulgating "The Culture of Martial Arts" and commanded General Dewa to summon several dozen of the lower level Samurai and have them train martial arts.[44] Minister of Finance Goto Shinpei said, The first step in self-

---

[42] Japanese Crown Prince Hirohito 裕仁 (1901–1989)

[43] *At 1:30 His Majesty arrived in Shuri. Taking pictures with his own camera, the crown prince enjoyed the event. He then climbed the steps up to Shuri Castle and watched Judo and Kendo duels prepared for his majesty. There was also a demonstration of Karate. (This is a digression, but His Majesty appeared to be extremely interested in Karate. The following year he invited the overall director Funakoshi Gichin to the royal palace to do a demonstration there. This was the key event that propelled Karate's expansion across Japan.)*

Homeland and Youth 祖国と青年
By Megumi Ryunosuke 惠隆之介 (1954~)
June 1986

[44] Shogun Yoshimune 徳川吉宗 (1684 ~1751) was appalled that many Samurai seemed unable to ride a horse or even swim. He ordered more training and large-scale hunting parties.

cultivation is correcting your mind and being sincere.[45] Marquise Ogasawara referred to Karate as "A technique of divine elegance." General Affairs Director Takejiro described it as, "Parting the clouds, seeking the way obscured."[46] General Hishikari described Karate as "Barehanded Karate For Defense of the Entire Body." [47] Rear Admiral Kanna wrote his opinion on adding Karate to the fitness regimen aboard navy ships and submitted it to the department of the Navy. General Oka wrote, "Following the war this is an excellent resource for the Japanese people education." Researcher Higashionna describes Karate as "The martial art of men of virtue."

---

[45] Count Goto Shinpei　後藤新平　　　(1857 ~ 1929)
Physician and cabinet minister
[46] Tokonami Takejiro　床次竹二郎　　(1866 ~ 1935)
Cabinet minister
[47] Takashi Hishikari　　菱刈隆　　　(1871 ~ 1952)
徒空手連体護身

Yomiuri Newspaper
Wednesday, October 8th 1924

Big Karate Brawl, Three Ryukyu Men Seriously Injured

に文目月用会の改正案について審
譲する筈

唐手で突合ひ
琉球人大怪我

（横濱電話）六日午前十一時半頃横濱市中村町一三一六沖繩生れ喜敷驫喜（二五）方で同縣人の渡嘉敷晴（二三）赤峰鑑人（二〇）の三名が飲中些細のことから口論を始め何れも沖繩特有の唐手を以て突き合ひ三名共胸部顔面血等に何れも二三週間を要する打撲傷を負ふた

Yomiuri Newspaper
Wednesday, October 8th 1924

Big Karate Brawl, Three Ryukyu Men Seriously Injured

At 11 pm on October 6th in front of No. 136 Naka-machi, Yokohama City, three Ryukyu men, Kiyabu Kamekichi (25,) Tokeshi Kameharu (23) and Akamine Kaneto (26) were out drinking when a trivial matter resulted in an argument.

All three began fighting using Karate,[48] which is a martial art particular to Okinawa prefecture. The men struck each other in the face and chest. Bruises and other injuries are expected to take two to three weeks to heal.

---

[48] Karate is written 唐手 "Chinese Hand" with the reading Karate.

日本之醫界
The Nippon Medical World
July 1926

東大醫科

◇唐手會組織さる　琉球拳法

唐手は「唐手に先手なし」と云ふ語がある如く、文明的護身術としては我柔道にも優つたものであると云ふので、醫學部三年の松田君、四年の檜君その他數君が發起となり、唐手會を組織し柔道部の諒解を得て、同部道場を借り、斯道の名手富名腰義珍氏を聘し、來る九月から練習を開始すると。

Tokyo University Medical School
Formation of a Karate Club

Ryukyu Kenpo Karate has a well-known saying, "Karate never makes the first strike" and this reflects the fact that it is a very cultured method of self-defense. It is a refined art on par with Judo, which was also developed in Japan. The club is being started by third grade medical student Matsuda and fourth year Himono[49]

Having reached an understanding with the Judo club, the Karate club will be using the same Dojo for training. A Mr. Funakoshi Gichin, an expert in this method, has been invited to be the instructor for the club, which will start in September.

---

[49] Himono Kazumi 檜物一三
Matsuda Shoichi 松田勝一

Ryukyu Meibutsu Karate no Hanashi
A Brief Introduction to Karate, the Famous Product of Ryukyu
By Sasaki Shoma 佐々木彰磨
Weekly Asahi　週間朝日
September 11th 1927

琉球名物 唐手術の話

佐々木彰麿

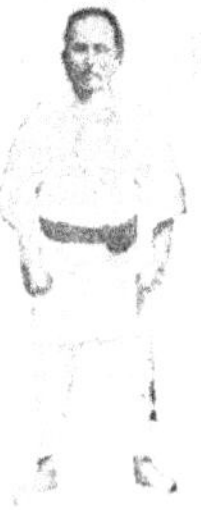

人道の手臨
富名腰義珍氏

へ掛の手臨

◇踏躍人の慣場

◇踏躍と手臨術

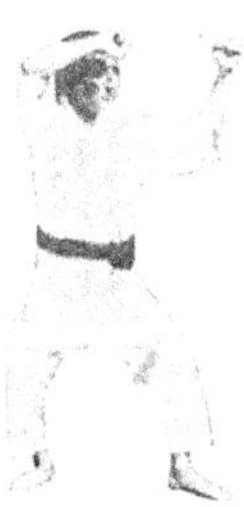

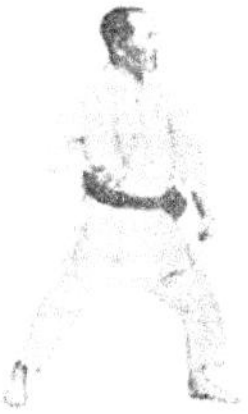

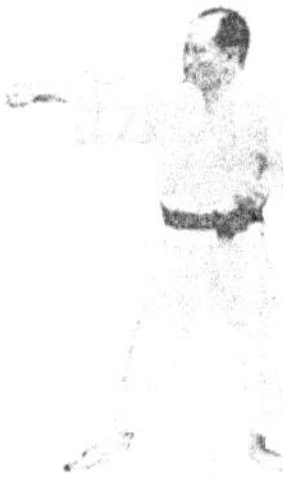

◇恐しい膂力

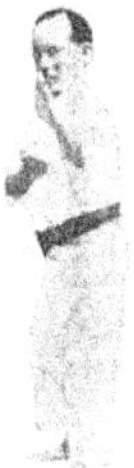

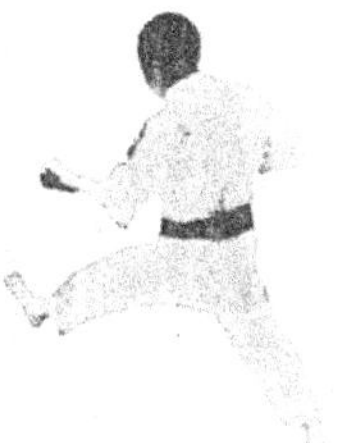

◇立論な護島術

◇隊手の車屋

◇誰も皆天覧を喜ぶ

◇今や東洋各國に

（をはり）

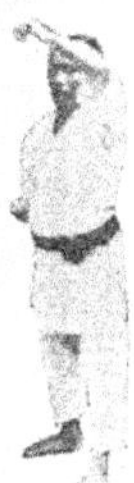

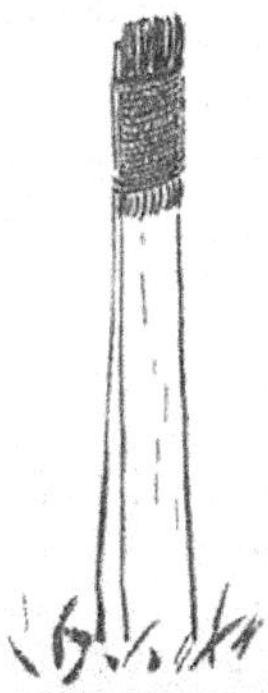

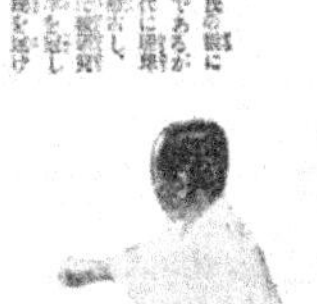

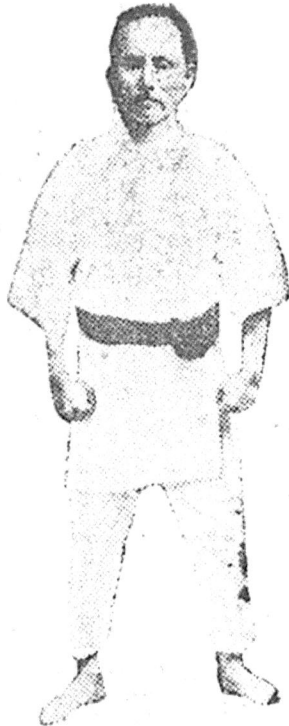

琉球名物

唐手術の話

唐手の達人

富名腰義珍氏

Karate no Tatsujin Funakoshi Gichin Shi
Karate Expert Mr. Funakoshi Gichin

A Brief Introduction to Karate, the Famous Product of Ryukyu
By Sasaki Shoma
September 11th, 1927

I can't recall exactly when, but a few days back I was reading a certain Tokyo newspaper and on the third page there was a story with the headline *Ryukyu men and Korean men get in a fight!*

Before I even read the story, the headline alone got me, *Ha ha ha! I already know the Ryukyu guys won!*

Reading the article, it turns out that several Ryukyu men and Korean men were all drinking together when an argument broke out. The Koreans had knives but the Ryukyu men didn't have so much as a Suntetsu, grappling spike.[50] All they had to face off against their opponents were their fists, yet the Ryukyu men left the Koreans bruised and battered, just as I predicted at the outset. The reason is because I know of the frightening martial from the Ryukyu archipelago, a mysterious martial art known as Karate Jutsu.

Not all Ryukyu people train Karate Jutsu, however many are intrinsically aware of the fundamentals of this art. I would like to take the time to explain a little about the famous martial art Karate (a type of Kenpo Jutsu, boxing.) [51]

While I mentioned that Karate is a type of boxing, it is nothing at all like the boxing you see in America or Europe. Starting fairly recently, European and American boxing events are being held

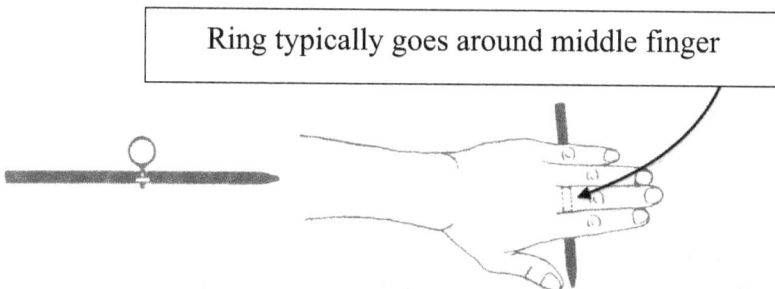

Ring typically goes around middle finger

50 Illustration of a Suntetsu, grappling spike. Typically, these were an iron rod pointed on one end and a ring in the middle. Either end could be used to press into vital areas and the flat side could be used to strike down onto any weapon an opponent might be holding. The saying, "Not armed with so much as a Suntetsu" appears frequently in old Jujutsu, Judo and Karate manuals.

51 Brackets are by the author.

regularly in Japan. In fact, the matches are quite popular. Just this past June the student boxing association and others formed the Japan Boxing Federation.

Further, on this past July 21st at Yankee Stadium in New York, there was a bout between the former World Boxing Champion Jack Dempsy and the rising challenger Bob Sharkey.[52] The electronic broadcast of that match inflamed the youth of Japan.

While European and American boxing is becoming all the rage, there is a fantastic style of *Kento Jutsu Karate*, Karate Boxing, that has been around in our country for two hundred years. Despite this there are no doubt many people, who despite being Japanese, are not aware of this. Truthfully, it is not all that surprising that people don't know about Karate as it is only practiced on one island in the Ryukyu archipelago, way to the south of Kyushu. However, nowadays Karate Jutsu is becoming popular in Tokyo, and is growing rapidly, but I will discuss that later.

Karate Jutsu is a style of boxing unique to Ryukyu and is referred to locally as Tekubushi. Tekubushi refers to hands and fists. Practitioners of this art are able to crush their opponents and defend themselves despite being barehanded and not armed with so much as a Suntetsu.

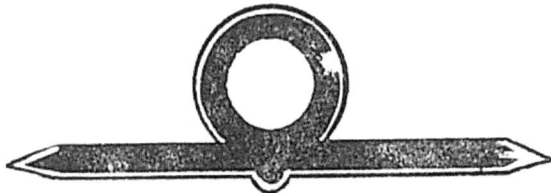

寸鉄

Illustration of a Suntetsu

There are many secret methods in Karate Jutsu. Just like there are Dojo in Kendo, Karate practitioners in Ryukyu train in Dojo. When training, expert instructors will train diligently with each and every student, to ensure they understand.

---

[52] Dempsey knocked out Bob Sharkey in the seventh round before 80,000 fans.

Karate Jutsu to Kento Jutsu
Karate versus Boxing

As for the differences between Karate and boxing, in European and American boxing they follow the Queensbury Rules. Thus, both combatants wear gloves and striking is limited to the upper body. Further, gripping the upper body like in Sumo is forbidden. In Karate there are no such restrictions. In Karate both the hands and feet are used in conjunction. Typically, the hands strike, the feet kick and the target is primarily the chest, groin and stomach, extending out to the sides where the kidneys are. Practitioners target Kyusho, vital areas, like the face, nose, cheeks, temples, jaw and so on. In addition, there are throws like Neji Taushi, Tani Otoshi, Yari Tama, Kubiwa, Nodo Osae, much like in Judo, therefore it is quite dangerous.

As striking a vital area can lead to a fatal injury, Karate is not something that can be turned into a competitive sport for entertainment like European and American boxing. Karate is fundamentally not an appropriate martial art to put on display in front of spectators. Currently there is some experimenting to see if it would be possible to have Karate matches where both combatants wear protective gear and with the understanding that Kyusho, vital points, are off limits to kicks and punches, but this seems a difficult proposition to me. Recently there have been frequent attempts to pit Judo against Karate, however as they realized how dangerous it was, the matches were stopped. Recently people have frequently tried to arrange Judo versus boxing matches, but as such a bout would be dangerous, the plans were abandoned. As difficult as finding a way to conduct a Judo versus boxing match may be, finding a way to hold a Judo versus Karate match is infinitely more difficult.

Unfortunately, the only way to see a Karate bout is if you happen to be around when two practitioners get into a fight and really go at it. If you would like to see Karate Kata however, is possible to see several of them. If you happen to see a demonstration of Karate Kata you will be amazed at how developed the practitioners' bodies are. Their kicks and punches flash out vigorously.

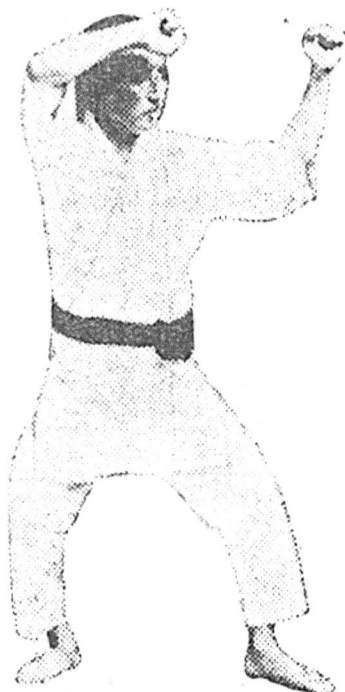

唐 手 の 構 へ

Karate no Kamae He
Going into Karate Kamae

A Fearful Level of Power

In order to improve striking power and toughen their fists, Karate Jutsu practitioners use a Makiwara. This is shown in the illustration. If you see the hands of a Karate Jutsu practitioner, you will notice their knuckles have developed stunningly to the point that they are all black and rock hard. That fist striking an object would no doubt cause it to ring like a metal hammer striking a bell and hardly seems like something a person could endure.

Nowadays, any person who has trained Karate even a little bit can easily snap a half-inch board or crack a roof tile. There is the story of a certain man from Ryukyu who joined the navy and is said to have once struck an iron plate hard enough that it left a dent, much to the astonishment of the other students at the officer training school.

Further, recently at Tokyo Imperial University Dojo a certain student of the famous Karate Practitioner Funakoshi Gichin stacked up four boards that were 8/10ths of an inch thick on top of each other and struck them with his fist. The story goes, his punch spilt all four boards in spectacular fashion.

In the face of such power, it is clear that if you are hit by one punch from a Ryukyu man, you are unlikely to emerge alive. If you are struck by a Karate attack, while there won't be any sign of injury on the outside, you may have broken bones or ruptured organs. Such stories are frequently reported.

This ends the introduction of Makiwara training which is used to strengthen the power of the fist. However, if you wish to study Karate Jutsu seriously and advance until you understand the inner mysteries of the art, you will need a teacher.

A truly astonishing variety of methods are used in Karate to train and forge the body. A stack of rice straw bales full of sand are stacked chest high and Shisatsu Ho, Piercing Killing Method, using all five fingers striking simultaneously is trained. Grip strength is trained by squeezing thick pieces of green bamboo until they shatter. Practitioners are also taught how to jump forward and back in order to either attack or defend when faced with an opponent, how to defend against a spear or sword, how to use a Bo as well as how to toughen the body and train the muscles of the chest, lower abdomen and back. There are innumerable such training methods.

Once you have become adept at these techniques, to the average person you will seem extraordinary. There are many people who can demonstrate these amazing techniques. For example, some can, from a seated position, leap up and kick off the ceiling, rip beef apart barehanded, crack green bamboo with their grip, punch through five or six half-inch thick boards stacked up. They can grip the ceiling beams of a roof and climb along and do Sankaku Tobi (this is a triangular jump. You jump from the first point towards the second point, but before your feet land on the second point you switch the direction you are facing. Finally, you jump to the third point.)[53] These and others are all famous stories from great martial arts practitioners from the past.

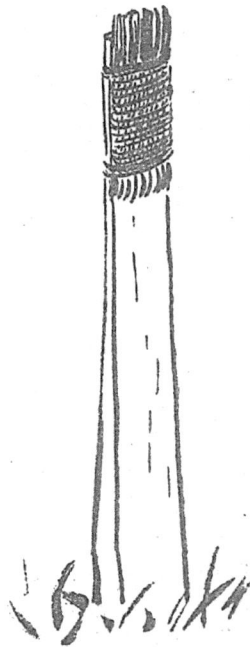

巻藁の圖 衝く練習拳を慣らす爲めに用ふ。杭の全長約七尺で地上四尺五寸、地下二尺五寸、幅三寸、厚さ上端五分、下端二寸五分、突く度に弾力ある様に出來てゐる。

Makiwara Illustration

This is for striking practice in order to condition the fist. Find a stake about seven feet tall and bury it two and a half feet in the ground so about four and a half feet are sticking up. It should be about three inches thick. The upper portion should be five inches thick and the lower two and a half inches thick. When you strike it there should be some spring.

---

[53] Brackets are by the author.

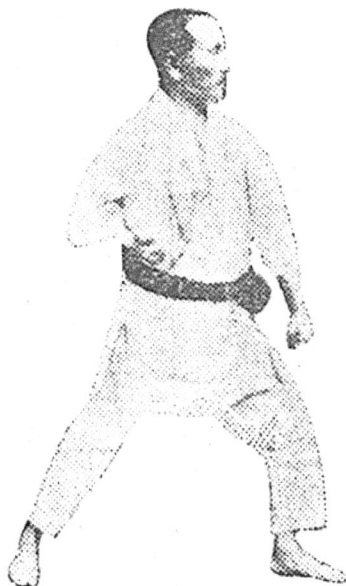

敵が丸腰や下腹部を
蹴って來たこころを
左手で受けて右
が用意をしてゐる。

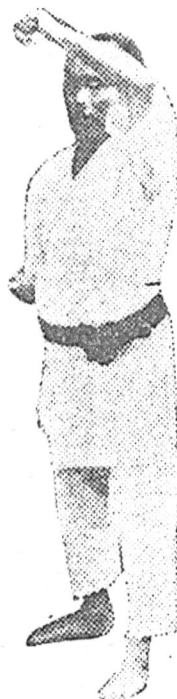

敵から顔面の攻撃を
受けたのを左手で受
けこめ右手は攻撃の
用意をしてゐる。

Left: When your opponent attacks your groin or lower abdomen, block with your left hand and prepare to strike with your right.

Right: When your opponent tries to punch you in the face, use your left hand to block and ready a strike with your right fist.

History of Karate

So, when exactly did the martial art of Karate come to Ryukyu? Karate is, as the Kanji in the word suggest, from China. China was long ago known as Kara, referring to the Tang dynasty, which existed from 618~907 AD. Thus, one prevailing theory is that the martial art was transmitted from China.

A certain oral tradition states that about two-hundred years ago a man known only as Sakugawa went to China to train and when he returned to Ryukyu, he spread what he had learned. There was also a Chinese man named Kusanku who taught what he knew on a trip to Ryukyu. There is another theory that when Ryukyu became a vassal state of Satsuma Domain in the fourteenth year of Keicho, weapons were banned and had to be handed in to officials. Due to this it seems likely the people had no choice but to develop an unarmed method of combat.

However, the greatest Karate practitioner alive today, Mr. Funakoshi Gichin, has the most likely scenario. According to Mr. Funakoshi, Karate is a weapon unique to Ryukyu. During an era when the people of Ryukyu worshiped everything Chinese, Ryukyu people began training Chinese martial arts. Then they began adding elements of Chinese martial arts to the native martial arts of Ryukyu, and the end result was a new martial art that took the best from Chinese martial arts. They even took the Kanji Kara and added it to "Te," method, and thereby creating "Kara-te."
I personally agree with this explanation.

If you ever see two Ryukyuan people fighting, even a person unfamiliar with Karate, will be able to understand that they don't have any tradition of carrying around bladed weapons. They only use their fists to strike each other. Even fights among children are intense, and make the fights between children in other prefectures look quite tame in comparison. The reason is they swing using Tekken, Iron Fist Strikes. Even if the children don't actually study Karate, it is remarkable that they still attack each other in Karate Shiki, Chinese Hand Fashion.

下通の流人
同輩の者集り
したゝかに呑み
又は喧嘩する事
如此、多く此類
流人なり。
ばくえき酒乱は
流人の常と知る
べし。

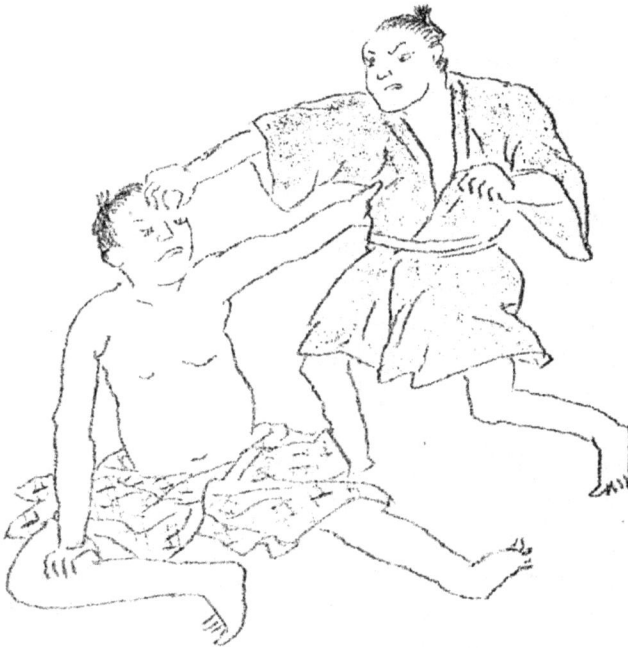

When lower class Ryukyu men get together, they often drink and fight. When the fight it looks like the picture. This is what a lot of the Ryukyu people are like. Gambling and drunkenness are a feature of the Ryukyu people.

-*Nanto Zatsuwa* 南島雑話
Tales From the Southern Isles
1855

A Splendid Method of Self-Defense

At present Karate has been added to the curriculum at Okinawa Junior High Schools. The schools teach only Karate Kata and not practical applications of the techniques. As for how Karate came to be taught in schools, there is an interesting episode[54] that explains this.

The story is, from days long past all Karate masters kept their style of Karate secret as they didn't want outsiders to find out about it. Thus, they trained their students in strict secrecy, that is until around the 34th ~35th year of Meiji. That was when the surprising results of a physical examination of youth was conducted and some were found to be surprisingly well-developed. The researchers found that the youths with bodies in the best condition had been training Karate. Realizing the positive effects, a Karate course was added to Junior High Schools and teacher training schools.

If you were to train Karate for a year, it would transform your entire body. That being said, just a few short months of training would create a striking difference that would distinguish you from average people. Thus, Karate Jutsu can be thought of not only as an excellent method of self-defense but also an extremely valuable as a way to improve physical fitness.

Famous Karate experts from Ryukyu all lived long lives. This includes the Elder Gentleman Itosu lived to be eighty-six, the Elder Gentleman Asato lived to be eighty-one, both Elder Gentleman Yamaguchi and Chinen who lived to be eighty-six, both Elder Gentleman Chihana and Zakihara who lived to be eighty and the Elder Gentleman Kiyuna who lived to be seventy-five. This seems to indicate that Karate training contains some sort of secret medicine that puts young men who don't train to shame. You could probably pit twenty men against each of these masters and have no effect. It seems that Karate training is what has allowed them to live such long lives.

---

[54] The author uses the English word "episode."

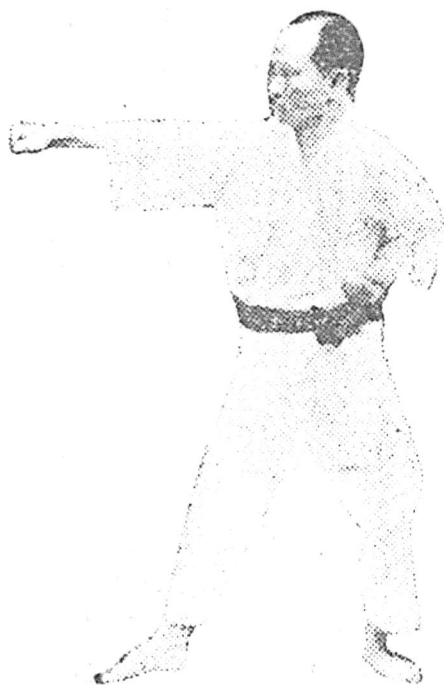

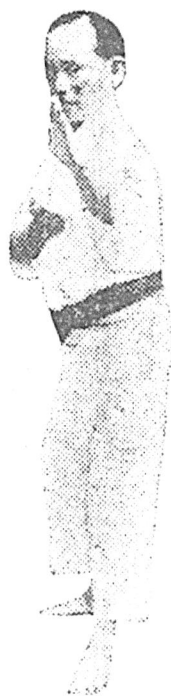

敵の攻撃手に樺
へながら敵を指
で刺殺せんこす
る勇姿。

こけ受で手右を撃攻の敵

は襲を敵が手の左や今め

るゐてしこん

Left: Block your opponent's strike with your right hand and ready your left hand to attack your opponent.

Right: Position after you have swept your opponent's strike aside and are attacking with a powerful Shisatsu, Piercing Killing strike

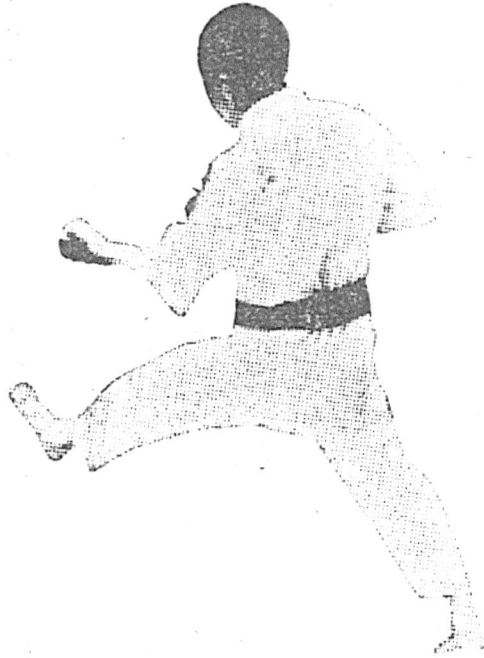

同こるけ受で手左を撃攻の敵
の丸睪の敵じ乗に隙の敵に時
は拳の左は俏 。る蹴をりたあ
。るへ横に撃攻

After blocking your opponent's strike with your left hand you immediately use that opening to kick in the area around your opponent's groin. Your left fist is ready to strike.

Blessed to Have Demonstrated Before the Emperor

While His Majesty the Emperor resides in the Imperial Palace in Tokyo, in March of the tenth year of Taisho (1921) went on an overseas excursion. At His Majesty's first port of call, he viewed a demonstration of Karate, that famous product of Ryukyu. It is reported that His Majesty was impressed at the demonstration and enjoyed it thoroughly. Further, when Prince Chichibu[55] was travelling to the United Kingdom, he too made a brief stop in Ryukyu, where he enjoyed a Karate demonstration. More and more the spotlight is shining on Ryukyu Karate.

In addition, people like Admiral Dewa and the late Admiral Murakami Hikonojoboth visited Ryukyu and observed Karate demonstrations while in port at Nakagusuku Bay. The first time was with the First Imperial Fleet and later when Yashuiro Rokuro was Admiral in charge of the Second Imperial Fleet. [56] The admirals commented that Karate seemed an appropriate martial art for sailors to learn.

In particular Admiral Yashuiro had a deep understanding of Karate and, every morning while his ships were in port, went out of his way to send sailors to the junior high school to train Karate. Whenever famous people visit Ryukyu, they are taken to seen the famous Karate demonstrations and, invariably, they are impressed by the masculine performance.[57]

---

[55] Prince Chichibu (1902 ~ 1953) was the second son of the Taisho Emperor and a younger brother of Hirohito.

[56] Admiral Dewa Shigeto   出羽重遠   (1856 ~ 1930)

Admiral Kamimura Hikonojo   上村彦之丞   (1849 ~ 1916)

Yashiro Rokuro   八代六郎   (1860 ~1930)

[57] Map on the following page shows Nakagusuku Bay from General Map of Ryukyu 廻七拾四里 Edo Era

Nakagusuku Bay

Now In the Eastern Capital

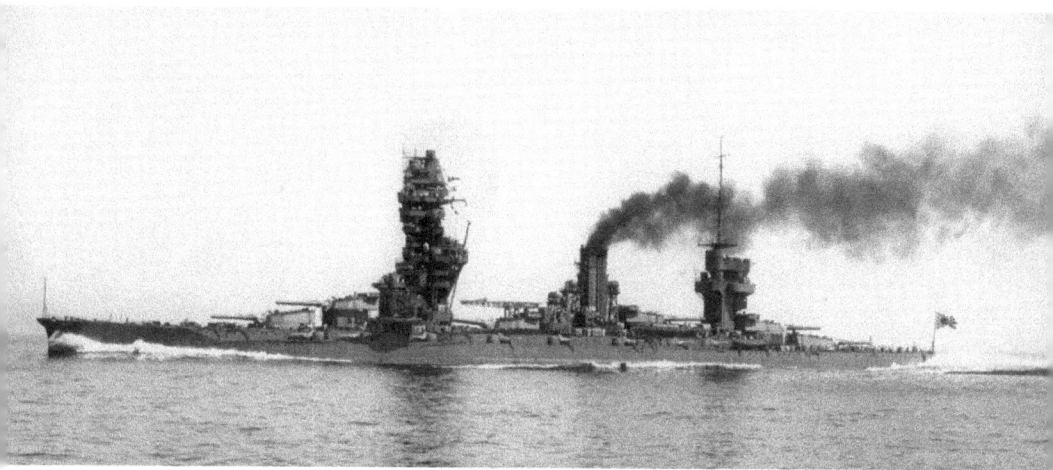

Battleship Fuso
Launched 1914, sunk in the Battle of Surigao, October 25th 1944

When Rear Admiral Kanna was captain of the Japanese battleship Fuso [58] he was of the opinion that Karate was an essential martial art for soldiers. He submitted a proposal that Karate be taught generally, even going so far as to include pictures of how the techniques should be performed. Apparently, the plan was rejected as other officers felt that if hot tempered young men began fighting using Karate after drinking alcohol, it could lead to a dangerous situation where Karate was used to cause trouble. However, I don't think that is a concern.

The problem is that a great many people don't know anything about Karate or they hallucinate that it is some ancient, primitive martial art and crassly dismiss it. I don't believe there is another martial art that is as refined and gentlemanly as Karate. Nowadays when people are free to carry about all manner of weapon, some question if it is really necessary to learn an unarmed combat system to defend yourself and break your attacker. However, nowadays with many people clamoring about women's virtue, training Karate would give women and girls a perfect method of self-defense.

---

[58] Kanna Kenwa 漢那憲和 (1877~ 1950)

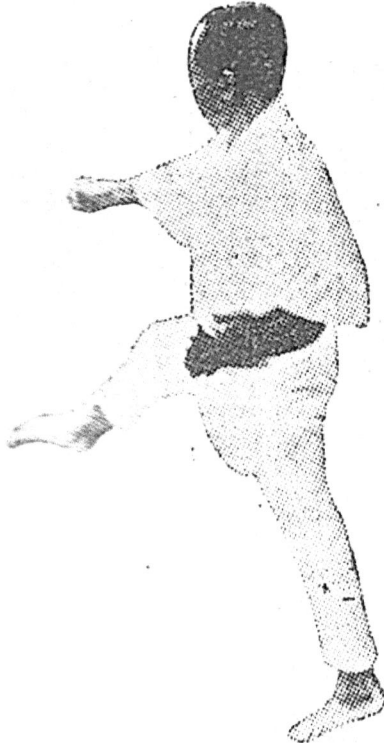

の右をこさた來てつ打の敵
左り敵で足に共さるけ受で手
霊を敵てめ固を拳に正は手の
るゐてし意用さんか

When your opponent attacks, block with your right hand and, at the same time, kick. Your right hand is ready in a fist to attack if needed.

So then, in conclusion, of late Karate Jutsu has, through good fortune and timing, travelled from a lonely island in the southern seas to the flower of Tokyo. The great martial arts practitioner and educator Kano Jigoro Sensei of the Kodokan has a thorough understanding of this art. Karate is already being taught at the Toyama Army Academy. Currently Karate master Funakoshi Gichin is instructing dedicated students at Tokyo Imperial University as well as Keio University. Just a few days ago, I took it upon myself to visit the Imperial University and there I saw dozens of Imperial University students training with gusto.

According to Mr. Funakoshi, he does have one female student. While Karate is of course beneficial for men, women can use Karate to strengthen their bodies and by learning it they also equip themselves with a method of self-defense.

End

Yomiuri Newspaper
December 4th 1932

Karate Jutsu no Kyogika
The Sportification of Karate Jutsu

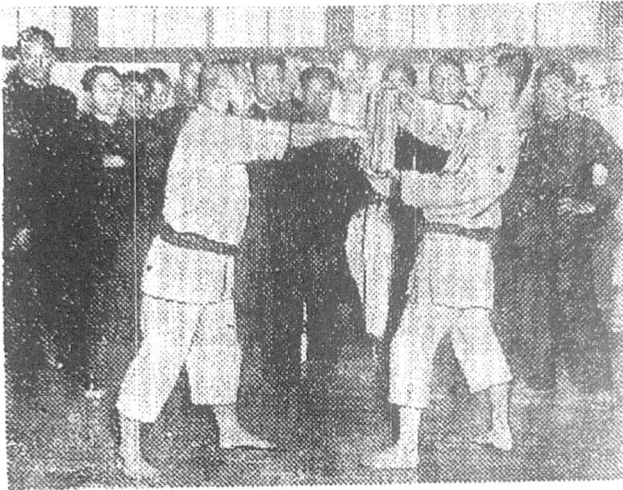

唐手術の競技化
一般人命を戦ひつ「唐手」は今まで試合の
不可能の状態にあつたつがれば思とのもるす達變び呼を味　ら
寶の初最日三はで究研大東がれは思とのもるす達變び呼を味
演實「割板」の氏池小範師大洋東は眞寫、たつ行に場道大東を會演

Yomiuri Newspaper
December 4th 1932

Karate Jutsu no Kyogika
The Sportification of Karate Jutsu

Up until now Karate, which can kill a person with a single blow, did not have any competitions. However recently dueling pads have been developed. This will no doubt be popular with spectators. On December 3rd the Tokyo University Karate Training Club held its first demonstration match at the Tokyo University Dojo.

The picture is of Tokyo university Karate instructor Koike doing Ita-wari, board breaking.

Recalling the Past Decade
By Funakoshi Gichin
From Mabuni Kenwa's *Karate Kenpo The Art of Self-Defense* 1934

十年前の回顧

富名腰義珍

摩文仁賢和君は私の竹馬の友で、近世稀に見る空手研究家で、現在の専門家中錚々たる者である。嘗て郷里にゐた頃は、縣下同好の士を集め、君は首里で、私は那覇で、各々會を組織して互に青年子弟を勵まし、殆ど寢食を忘るると云ふ風な、不眠不休の體であつた。

次ぎから次ぎと、傳へ聞いて馳せ參ずる者多く晝夜門人の出入絶えなかつた。

君は溫行篤實な君子人で未だ曾て流派の爭等は微塵も念頭に置かず、知らざる

Recalling the Past Decade
By Funakoshi Gichin
An introduction to Mabuni Kenwa's *Karate Kenpo The Art of Self-Defense* 1934

Mabuni Kenwa has been my friend since the days when we used to play on bamboo stilts. Of late, he has become the focus of attention as a Karate practitioner and researcher, and indeed is considered the eminent expert in this field. When he was living in our homeland, many of us Karate practitioners from the same prefecture would gather together. Though he was from Shuri and I was from Naha and each of us had our own organizations, we still each encouraged the students of the other. At that time, we rarely remembered to sleep or eat, and we worked ourselves to the bone.

One after another people began to hear of what we were doing and Karate disciples were coming and going all day and all night with no end in sight. Mabuni is a *Kunshi*, martial arts gentleman, with a gentle and sincere personality. If he ever found out about a certain fighting technique in some branch of Karate he relentlessly pursued any information about it, asking all practitioners, irrespective of whether they were his *Senpai* (先輩, "senior") or his *Kohai* (後輩, "junior.")

Ever polite and humble he would bow his head and ask for information.

Later, having learned the new technique, he would not simply keep it to himself but readily share it with everyone at the next available chance. This is so we could all research the technique together. His philosophy of sharing all the information he found was completely the opposite of the old way of doing things, where everything was kept secret.

After collecting materials for a long time, there is no doubt that Mabuni Kenwa possesses the greatest amount of material related to Karate and knows the most techniques. This fact alone makes it clear referring to him as *first under heaven* (unparalleled in his field) is not an exaggeration. Upon occasion a joint Embu, public martial arts demonstration, would be held by neighboring Naha and Shuri Karate Dojo. If Mabuni received any criticism, he listened and immediately went about correcting the issue. Further, whenever he watched other schools, he offered critiques that highlighted the strengths and supplement any shortcomings. A critique done with the feeling of mutual consideration. Everyone is interested in what he has to say and he is highly regarded. You will never find a critic or someone who attacked him.

Recently, I hear Mabuni Kenwa has gone to Osaka and has redoubled his efforts teaching young students. This is not only at Kansai University but also in the surrounding area. His goal in the end is to teach people about Karate for the country and for society. I am thrilled that of late he has found success and the rave reviews he is receiving in the Kansai area only confirms this. Next, he seeks to join east to west and establish a unified overall network and I am pleased beyond words at this development.

Of late Mabuni Kenwa has become a writer and he asked me to write something for him, in response to that I have recorded my recollections here to the best of my ability.

Confucius Sayeth;

A great person is one who does not speak a lot, but takes care to make his actions nimble.

Confucius (480~350 BC)
From *The Analects*

Asahi Newspaper
October 30th 1936
Birth of the Student Karate Organization

Asahi Newspaper
October 30th 1936
Birth of the Student Karate Organization

For the past decade Funakoshi Gichin has been teaching Karate, based on the Karate Jutsu, which was developed in Ryukyu. In fact, it has become a sport taught at many schools. Already there are All Japan Student Karatedo Organizations at Waseda, Keio, Taku, Ho, Sho and Ichiko. The president of the new organization will be Saigo Yoshinosuke. An event celebrating the founding of the organization will be held Aoyama Hall on November 7th at 1pm.

Following the ceremony, the first public demonstration and competition will be held. Each school will be sending athletes to compete. Kata as well as Kumite and Shiai, duels, will be held.

Kento – Boxing
Joe Eagle vs Takasu Goro
Twelve Rounds
Otsu Masaichi vs Sakamoto Hajime
Five other bouts
Night of November 2nd
If rain, will be held the next day
Hibiya Concert Hall

Karatedo and the Japanese Spirit
Funakoshi Gichin
Pen Magazine
January 1937

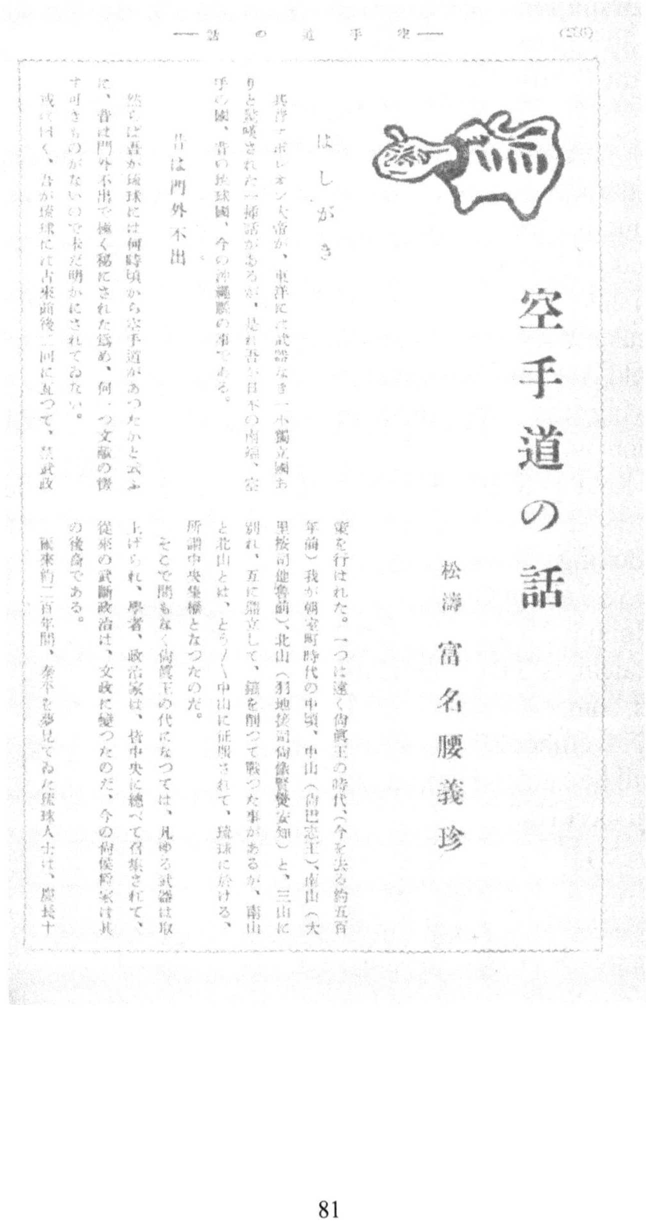

―空手道の話―

空手道の話

松濤　富名腰義珍

はしがき

其昔ナポレオン大帝が、東洋には武器なき一小獨立國ありと驚嘆された一挿話があるが、是れ吾が日本の南端、空手の國、昔の琉球國、今の沖繩縣の事である。

昔は門外不出

然らば吾が琉球には何時頃から空手道があつたかと云ふに、昔は門外不出で極く秘にされた爲め、何一つ文獻の徴す可きものがないので未だ明かにされてゐない。

或は曰く、吾が琉球には古來前後二回に亘つて、禁武政策を行はれた。一つは遠く尚眞王の時代（今を去る約五百年前）我が朝室町時代の中頃、中山（尚巴志王）、南山（大里按司他魯毎）、北山（羽地按司怕尼芝攀安知）と、三山に別れ、互に鼎立して、鎬を削つて戰つた事があるが、南山と北山とは、とう／＼中山に征服されて、琉球に於ける、所謂中央集權となつたのだ。

そこで間もなく尚眞王の代になつては、凡ゆる武器は取上げられ、學者、政治家は、皆中央に總べて召集されて、從來の武斷政治は、文政に變つたのだ。今の尚侯爵家は其の後裔である。

爾來約二百年間、泰平を夢見てゐた琉球人士は、慶長十

Karatedo and the Japanese Spirit
Funakoshi Gichin
Pen Magazine
January 1937

Karatedo, Past and Present

There's a story about the emperor Napoleon who was shocked to hear that there was a small country in the east where nobody had any weapons. The story was describing was the extreme southern portion of Japan, the nation of Karate long ago called Ryukyu nowadays known as Okinawa Prefecture.[59]

---

[59] With the exception of a momentary fit of scorn and incredulity when told the Loo-Chooans (Ryukyuans) had no wars or weapons of distraction, he [Napoleon] was in high good humour while examining me on these topics. The cheerfulness, I may almost call it familiarity, with which he conversed, not only put me quite at ease in his presence, but made me repeatedly forget that respectful attention which it was my duty, as well as my wish on every account, to treat the fallen monarch.

- Interview With Buonaparte
Basil Hall (1788 ~ 1844)

Interestingly, Hall discussed Okinawa with Napoleon himself when the Lyra put in at St. Helena, and reported in his account that:
Several circumstances ...respecting the Loo-Choo (Ryukyu) people surprised even him a good deal; and I had the satisfaction of seeing him more than once completely perplexed, and unable to account for the phenomena I related. Nothing struck him so much as their having no arms. "Point d'armes!" he exclaimed... "Mais, sans armes, comment se bat-on?"

I could only reply, that as far as we had been able to discover, they had never had any war, but remained in a state of internal and external peace. "No wars!" cried he, with a scornful and incredulous expression, as if the existence of any people under the sun without wars was a monstrous anomaly.

-George H. Kerr
Okinawa: The History of an Island People 1958

The origins of Karate are thought to date back to Keicho 14 (over three hundred years ago) when Lord Shimazu defeated Ryukyu and then commanded that all weapons be collected and their use banned. In response, Okinawan Samurai developed a method of unarmed combat to defend themselves called *Mutekatsu Ryu Karate*, Winning Without a Weapon School of Karate.[60]

Thus, it came to pass that for centuries in Okinawa Prefecture, Karate was always practiced in extreme secrecy. The rules regarding training groups were so strict that you couldn't even tell your own parents, brothers or sisters anything about what you were doing. It goes without saying that there were no official Dojo, rather we would practice at night in a room at our teacher's house and we would always finish training before the light of dawn.

It is completely unlike the training today that has seasonal special programs like Kangeiko, winter training, and training available at different times of the day. If the sky to the east began to brighten, we immediately had to stop training, eat breakfast and begin our studies. That was the way training was done every day of the year back then. It goes without saying that students from our school were not able to go and see what students from other schools were doing, and vice versa.

To give a sense of how strict the secrecy was, the overall feeling was not, "Don't talk about Karate to anybody outside the people you train with" instead it was, "Don't talk to anybody about Karate, ever."

However, just over the past thirty years or so the path of Karate has developing and expanding in surprising ways. Nowadays, all the universities in the Eastern Capital[61] are competing to set up Karate clubs and all the students are absorbed in training. In addition, there are private groups being set up that are following in the steps of the university groups in developing their skills.

Recently, Karate practitioner Marquis Saigo formed the All-Japan Student Karatedo Federation and became its first president. At this point it would be embarrassing for any gentleman who considers himself to be a martial artist to not know what Karatedo is. Comparing this era to what was happening thirty years ago I almost can't believe the changes that have occurred.

---

[60] *Mu-te-Katsu-Ryu* 無手勝流 Empty-Handed-Victory-School. Can also refer to "Defeating your opponent without fighting."

[61] Referring to Tokyo, since it is to the east of Kyoto.

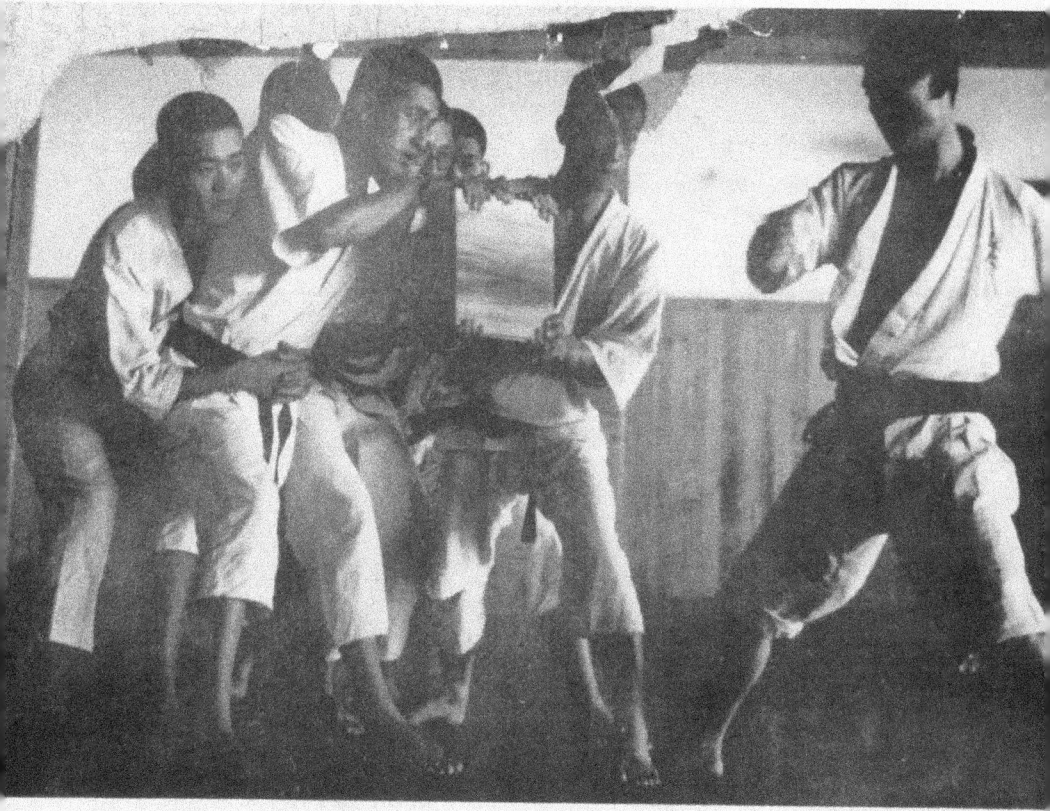

Tokyo University of Law Karate Club 1937
Ten board Ura Ken Tameshi Wari by club member Itoh Tomihide

Karatedo and Intellectual Training

Your typical person only receives intellectual training, book learning, while at school, however school is a place that teaches school rules and real learning doesn't happen until you've entered society. As the old saying accurately states, "You can't see the wide-open world from the window of a classroom." Once outside that system, you can look, feel and take in information from anywhere and everywhere.

For example, as Hong Zicheng says,

Once the true way has filled your mind, there will be no place for other desires to gain purchase.[62]

If your spirits is filled with the principles of justice, then intruding thoughts and desires cannot enter your mind.

---

[62] This line is a quote from the Caigentan 菜根譚 a compilation of aphorisms eclectically combines elements from the Three teachings (Confucianism, Daoism and Buddhism) Written by Hong Zicheng 洪自誠 in 1590.
The full quote:

心不可不虚、虚則義理来居、心不可不実、実則物欲不入
*You cannot allow your mind to be filled with a multitude of overlapping thoughts and desires. The only way to allow the true way to fill your spirit is to have a mind empty of distraction. **Once the true way has filled your mind, there will be no place for desire to gain purchase.***

Thinking of this in terms of Bushido, if your body is operating at its full capacity, then there is no way for an opponent's attack to reach you.

While walking down the road people will make way for one another, and farmers will be willing to shift the borders of their fields.[63]

If that were the case, you would have no complaints. However, if a person on the road does not make way for you, or a fellow farmer is not willing to adjust the border of his field, this will invariably lead to a collision. The reason is, each person has their own desires, and this results in conflict, both interpersonal and within society as a whole.

You can find innumerable similar examples anywhere you look. In Karatedo, to achieve the ultimate level, you must be able to change, transform and adapt not only when facing an opponent, but when you're out in society in general.

Sometimes you will have to transform based on the time, sometimes you'll have to change based on the place and sometimes you will have to adapt based on the era you find yourself in. In short you must change, transform and adapt to the world around you.

---

[63] This quote is regarding an incident that happened during the reign of the King Wen of Zhou, China sometime around 1152~1050 BC. The countries of Gu 虞 and Zei 芮 were in the midst of a years-long dispute about farmlands and were unable to reach an accord. They decided to consult King Wen of Zhou(1152~1050 BC) as, "King Wen is a man of the highest caliber, he can tell which of us is correct."

The Kings of Gu and Zei went to King Wen's lands. They saw that the farmers were willing to shift the borders of fields in order to accommodate neighbors and peasants would step aside and allow others to pass on the road. In town, women and men walked separate from each other and you never saw old people carrying heavy goods. At court those of the warrior class were deferential to elder advisors and the elder advisors were deferential to the government.

Karatedo and Moral Education

If you were to look at Karatedo and consider how it can foster the people of Japan's moral education, you would see that the base is formed by the same core of loyalty found in Bushido. In other words, a reverence for martial spirit, fidelity to one's principles, maintaining proper manners and etiquette, being a person of good faith, being generally humble, having a sense of honor, love of fellow man, being diligent, being able to endure, remaining unsullied, having persistence and a maintaining a daring spirit. These features are inherent in Karate, exactly like all other martial arts, and form inseparable bond to the nation and the very character of the Japanese people.

It goes without saying that martial arts and martial spirit are inextricably linked to humanity and justice and that, when teaching Karate, we explain it through the lens of humanity and teach that self-reflection is an essential part of duty. Should the need arise, the situation would be viewed from a humanist perspective and, in the end, the goal should be to reflect on where duty lies.

In short, those that train Karatedo do not actively seek out a fight, as the core philosophy is, *Karate practitioners do not make the first attack.* Yamaoka Tesshu also said something exactly in line with this philosophy, *The sword that offers no aid, the sword that will not cut.*[64]

It goes without saying that in Karate more emphasis is placed on defensive techniques than offensive and thus, from ancient times, it has been praised as a martial art for men of virtue, nay, a martial art for gentlemen. In fact, Karate is a martial art that fits perfectly not only with the Japanese mentality but also with contemporary culture.

Those of us who teach this art, frequently focus on *Shin Jutsu*, training mental fortitude, more than *Gi Jutsu*, training physical techniques. We focus on a person's inner nature rather than their outer

---

[64] Yamaoka Tesshu (1836~1888) a Samurai who played an important role in the Meiji Restoration. He was known for his knowledge of swordfighting, calligraphy and Zen. In an era when many Samurai were abandoning the way of the sword, Yamaoka became a fervent Kenjutsu practitioner. He felt that the way of the sword was not a method to kill people but to bring enlightenment to the self.

He is famous for his phrase *Kenzen Ichinyo* 剣禅一如 The way of the Sword and the way of Zen are one. The pinnacle of both Zen and the way of the sword are the same.

physical side. Rather than overwhelming an opponent through sheer power, we gain our opponent's respect by demonstrating our spiritual refinement.

We feel it is not only our civic duty, but our greatest mission to ensure that we are able to encourage the positive, healthy development of even one more citizen who is able to serve our nation.

Karatedo and Physical Education

The movements contained within Karatedo exercise all parts of your body and teach you how to move in every direction: forwards, backwards, to the left and to the right. You envision an opponent and train how to attack with your hands and feet in a particular way, against a particular spot. After long years of rigorously training this system, you will have undisputedly developed a fundamental understanding of the art.

In addition, this method evenly develops the various muscle groups in your face, neck, chest and stomach, in addition to teaching proper breathing, jumping ability as well as how to advance, how to retreat, move horizontally and diagonally. In short, this method develops all parts of your body equally and correctly in an organized fashion. Further, it is a streamlined method designed comprehensively develop your body in a state of harmony.

It is a fascinating art that once students begin, they find they can't quit along the way and, instead, must continue; truly a profound and mysterious art. The techniques are quite easy to memorize even after practicing them one time you can train them anytime and anyplace quite easily. In addition, anyone, man woman old or young can train this. And your body type doesn't matter either. It is a martial art that is not dangerous, doesn't require a lot of time and the only thing you need is a desire to participate. It is both a method of physical exercise as well as a method of self-defense, in addition it fosters mental development.

Karate can be thought of as the most effective method of rejuvenating your youth, as well as a method for living a long life as evidenced by the fact that nearly all the top practitioners in this art are well into their eighties, while simultaneously maintaining their vigor.

The Ability to Alternate Between Movement and Stillness

There is movement within stillness, there is stillness within movement. A core principle of the universe is that everything contains *Do-Sei*, both movement and stillness.[65] The arts of man follow the same principle, thus wise men of virtue, even when they are inactive must still possess the ability to respond in flesh should the need arise.

When thinking of this in terms of Karate, consider the situation where one hand has moved out to strike while the other is remaining quietly in reserve. In this case, the hand that you struck with can be considered Yang (Yo) while the resting hand can be thought of as Yin (In.)[66]

Another way to think of it as the striking hand is *Ki*, the unexpected attack, while your resting hand is *Sei*, the standard attack.[67] In short, when an opponent launches his first strike, the hand he holds in reserve should be considered significant and worthy of your attention. Understand that any fight exists somewhere between unexpected attack and traditional attack. The reason is, there are unexpected attacks that end up being straightforward attacks and, conversely, straightforward attacks that end up being unexpected attacks. If you are unable to adapt to this in a fight, then you will have a difficult time achieving victory. Often what is referred to as "mysterious" in a fight are these shifts between unexpected attacks and traditional attacks.

As for Kata, prescribed sets of movements, and Kamae, stances, those are simply steps on a ladder for you to follow in order to reach a natural state of enlightenment. It follows then that *Do-Sei*, movement and stillness, also does not represent the ultimate level. Not moving in order to be still, being still in order to not move, is not the goal. *Do-Sei* is the same as Yin-Yang, they should be thought of as how water forms into a wave. By unifying they become one, dividing them means there are two. Only by unifying *Do-Sei* can you achieve this.

---

[65] *Do-Sei* 動静 together the Kanji means "state of affairs" however in martial arts their meaning can be separated into "movement" and "stillness."

[66] The concept of Yin - Yang is very well-known in the West, however in Japan it is known as In-Yo.

[67] *Ki-Sei* 奇正 An unexpected attack versus A standard attack. A sneak attack versus A straight on attack.

Remember,
The superior man does not forget danger in his security [68]

There is an old philosophical warning that goes,

It is no good for a man to be knowledgeable only of the literary arts or to solely practice martial arts.[69]

Thus the people of Japan should always keep in mind that studying the literary arts and martial training are like the two wheels of a cart, or the two wings of a bird.

In times of peace, you cannot forget war, thus you should make forging your body a daily activity so that if there is a sudden crisis, we, as gentlemen are expected to respond to. At the same time the fact that your fellow countrymen will also respond is a beautiful characteristic of the Japanese.

Though the world seems to be at peace now with every nation chanting peace in unison, however, at the same time, as the current state of affairs shows, they are also building great warships,

---

[68] This is a quote from the *I Ching*. The full passage is as follows:

Danger arises when a man feels secure in his position. Destruction threatens when a man seeks to preserve his worldly estate. Confusion develops when a man has put everything in order. Therefore, the superior man does not forget danger in his security, not ruin when he is well established, nor confusion when his affairs are in order. In this way he gains personal safety and is able to protect the empire.
                              -Translated by Richard Wilhelm (1873 ~ 1930)
69

The Shiji 史記 *Records of the Grand Historian* 145~90 B.C by the Han dynasty historian Sima Qian. Records of the Grand Historian considered a "foundational text in Chinese civilization" covers the 2,500-year period from the age of the legendary Yellow Emperor to the reign of Emperor Wu of Han in the author's own time, and describes the world as it was known to the Chinese of the Western Han dynasty.

provisioning their armies and waiting like a crouching tiger for an opening[70] in an opposing country, what then is the point of it?

Karatedo and Kiai

The word *Kiai Jutsu* describes using your mind and spirit to battle the mind and spirit of your opponent. In this technique you are pitting your Seishin, will, against your opponent's will.

Looking at this from the perspective of psychology, Kiai Jutsu can be described as a state where you have focused all your mental energy on a single thing, compressing every ounce of your ability until it is like a beam of light directed at a single point.

From the perspective of philosophy, this method would be described as one that, utilizes the *Kyo-Jitsu*, total freedom to alternate between feints and true attacks, as well as Do-Sei, the unification and free use of movement and stillness.

From the perspective of Physiology, it is *Kokyu no Jutsu*, a method for regulating the breathing.

Finally, it can be simply described as *Kisaki wo Sei Suru*, stopping your opponent's attack before it even begins.

As far as examples of this technique being used, consider how Ito Ittosai used Musoken[71] to topple his opponent, or how Miyamoto Musashi used it to completely subdue Sasaki Ganryu, [72] Araki Mataemon faced off against Yagyu Munefuyu with nothing but a

---

[70] *Koshi Tantan* 虎視眈々 watching vigilantly like a tiger (for an opportunity to pounce)

[71] Ito Ittosai 伊藤 一刀斎 (1560 ~ 1653) The founder of the Itto School of Sword.

Musoken 夢想剣 reacting the moment your opponent launches his attack and moving in as you have completely anticipated your opponent's strategy.

[72] Sasaki Kojiro 佐々木小次郎 also known as Sasaki Ganryu (1585 ~ 1612) was defeated by Miyamoto Musashi in a duel on Boat Island in 1612.

white sheet of paper yet Munefuyu found himself unable to cut with his sword.[73] Other examples abound.

As for examples related to Karatedo, there is the emperor's aide-de-camp Nakamura, who was once suspended from duty for incurred the Imperial wrath[74] of the King of Ryukyu. Around that time a famous Karate practitioner named Uehara So-and-So [75] formally requested a duel. Matsumura, who at this point was ready to commit Seppuku, accepted Uehara's request, figuring that by throwing himself wholeheartedly into the duel, he would end up dying anyway.

That same total commitment of body and mind to the duel must have been apparent from the intent written on his brow as Uehara, despite his standing as a Karate expert, found himself paralyzed and unable to move his hands and feet. Though he made several attempts to engage with Matsumura, in the end he was forced to remove his helmet and admit defeat.[76]

---

[73] A duel between Araki Mataemon 荒木又右衛門 (1599~1638) and Yagyu Shinkage School sword master Yagyu Munefuyu 柳生宗冬 (1613－1675.) Mataemon was dueling the younger brother of his own sword master, Yagyu Jubei.

The duel began and Munefuyu took a stance armed with a wooden sword. However, Mataemon stood in Shodan Kamae, not with a wooden sword, but with a rolled-up piece of Japanese paper. Munefuyu found his opponent, despite being armed only with a sword of rolled up paper, had no weak points he could attack and admitted his defeat. This became known as *Boshi no Ken,* Sword Technique With Rolled Up Paper.

[74] *Genrin ni fureru* 逆鱗に触れる literally to rub scales in the wrong direction, meaning to incur the anger of your superior, generally referring to incurring the Imperial wrath.

[75] *Nanigashi* 某 a Kanji used in place of a person's name in order to maintain anonymity.

[76] *Kabuto wo Nugu* 兜を脱ぐ while it literally means "to remove your helmet" in this case it likely refers to "admitting superiority" or "to strike one's colors."

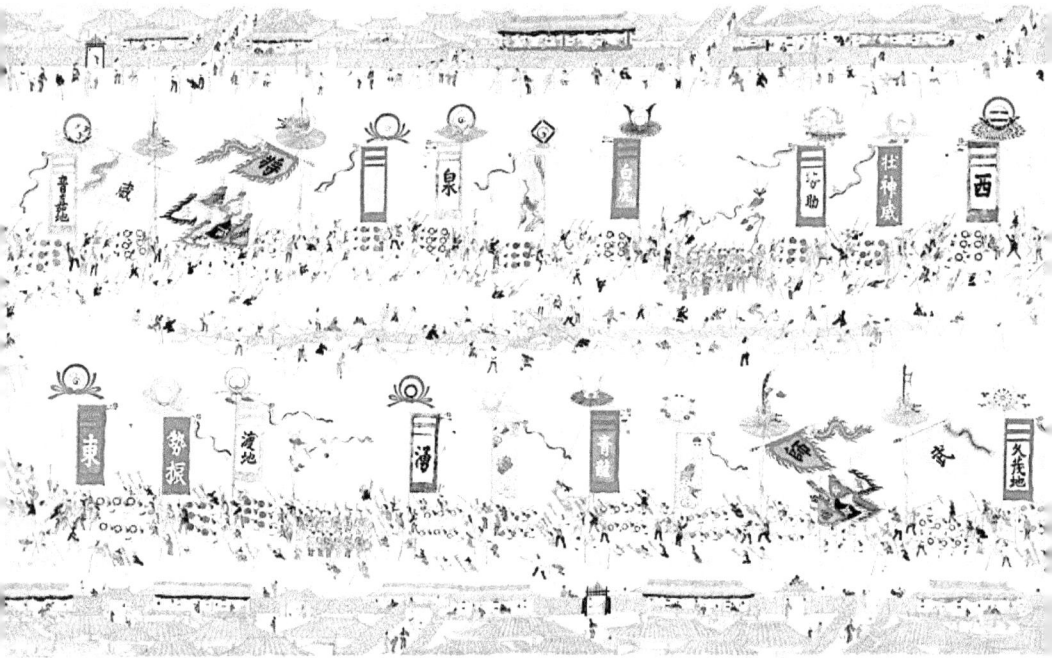

Illustration of the Naha City Tug of War
那覇四町綱之図
Date and artist unknown, 19th century

Also in Naha City, there was an annual tug of war event, and for some reason a great commotion had broken out that threatened to end in bloodshed. As the story goes, Higaonna Kanyu [77] (The revered father of Higashionna Kanjun [78] who is currently an instructor at Tokyo Prefectural High School) appeared on the scene and scolded the entire village with such fury that through the sheer force of his personality the attendees were all brought to submission and the event successfully concluded.

In Shuri City, there is a story about a man named Ishimine So-and-So was surrounded by a group of youths all carrying weapons. He neither became angry nor flustered but simply kept them at Bay by saying "Please wait a moment" before then finishing the meal he had been in the middle of. Having finished eating, he stood up, took a stance and breathed out with a sound like *Saa-Yoshi!* before saying, "OK then whoever's the strongest amongst you come at me!" The youths, who thought they had strength in their numbers, simply turned and left as they were overcome by his powerful force of presence.

All of these are examples of using Ki, your spirit, to control your opponent's Ki and thus can be thought of as examples of employing Kiai Jutsu, the art of using your force of presence to affect your opponent. A martial artist who, despite training, has not developed a understanding of this technique can hardly be said to be a true practitioner.

As Sun Tzu said in the Art of War, *Winning a hundred times in a hundred battles is not the ultimate achievement, the ultimate achievement is to defeat your enemy's soldiers without even joining battle.* It would be an error to think that this is not exactly what Aiki Jutsu describes.

---

[77] Higaonna Kanyu 東恩納 寛裕 （1849～1922） a Karate practitioner and government official active in the years before and after the Ryukyu Kingdom was absorbed into Japan.

[78] Higashionna Kanjun (東恩納 寛惇) also Higaonna Kanjun (14 October 1882 - 24 January 1963) was an Okinawan scholar who specialized in the history of Okinawa.

October 14th, 1939
Yomiuri Newspaper

Karatedo Demonstration and Competition
Athletes from Nine different universities participating, secret techniques to be revealed!

"空手道" 演武大會

九大學參加 祕技を公開

琉球に起源を發した拳法唐手術を日本武道化した空手道は最近各方面に普遍化され各大學専門校、會社商店等の研究團體が組織されてゐるが今春創設された關東學生空手道聯盟では十七日午後一時から切大記念館で演武大會を開催、東大、農大、立教、工大、日齒、日商、中大、慈惠、明大の加盟九校を始め京大も参加して祕技を公開する事となった

空手道は護身術として最も優秀なもので元來「突く、打つ、蹴る」の三法に「投げ、逆手、締め」の三法を加味し、効果的に身を守りよく敵を制する、併し決して闘爭の具とせず「侵さず侵されず」あくまで守るのを本義とし萬止むを得ざる危機に於て初めて活用されるもので體育的價値も大いに認められてゐる

October 14th, 1939
Yomiuri Newspaper

Karatedo Demonstration and Competition
Athletes from Nine different universities participating, secret techniques to be revealed!

Kenpo Karate Jutsu, which originated in Ryukyu but has now become a Japanese martial art, is now commonly practiced at universities and technical colleges all over Japan. Various companies and shops have also begun forming Karate practice groups.

The Kanto Regional Student Karatedo Organization which was formed this spring, will be hosting a demonstration and competition at Meiji University Anniversary Hall on October 17th at 1pm. Karate practitioners from Tokyo University, Tokyo Agricultural University, Tokyo Manufacturing University, Tokyo Medical University, Tokyo Dental University, Jikei University and Meiji University will participate. During the demonstration secret techniques will be shown.

Karatedo techniques are a highly effective method of self-defense. In addition to…

Tsuku – Thrust
Utsu – Strike
Keru – Kick

…which are the original Sanpo, Three Methods, the following have been added,

Nage – Throw
Gyakute – Joint Locks
Shime – Chokes

The addition of these means you can not only effectively defend yourself but also restrain an enemy, all without using any weapons or tools.

The fundamental principle of this art defensive, as demonstrated by the phrase, "Do not violate others, do not allow yourself to be violated." These techniques would only be applied if you were suddenly faced with a dangerous situation. Karate is widely viewed as being an effective method of physical education.

Regarding the Completion and Opening of the New Dojo
By Funakoshi Gichin
Head Instructor of the Shotokan
Karatedo Magazine Volume 3 Number 4
January 29ᵗʰ, 1939

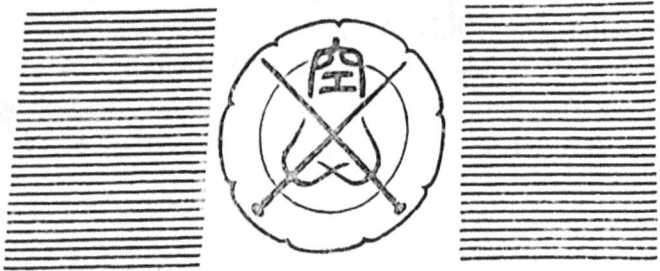

空 手 道

第 三 卷, 第 四 號

Regarding the Completion and Opening of the New Dojo
Funakoshi Gichin
Head Instructor of the Shotokan
January 29th, 1939

As the saying goes, "From days long past, a person that lives to be seventy is a rare person indeed." While I am approaching the "rare age of seventy" for those who train Karatedo, seventy years old is hardly a rare thing and I certainly plan on continuing to work to my fullest. Today, thanks to all of your support, we are celebrating the completion of a designated Dojo. While I am not sure what the rumors are saying regarding how this new Dojo compares to the ones in other martial arts traditions, what I can say is that this is the largest and most well-appointed Karatedo Dojo. Truly a rare thing in the history of Karatedo.

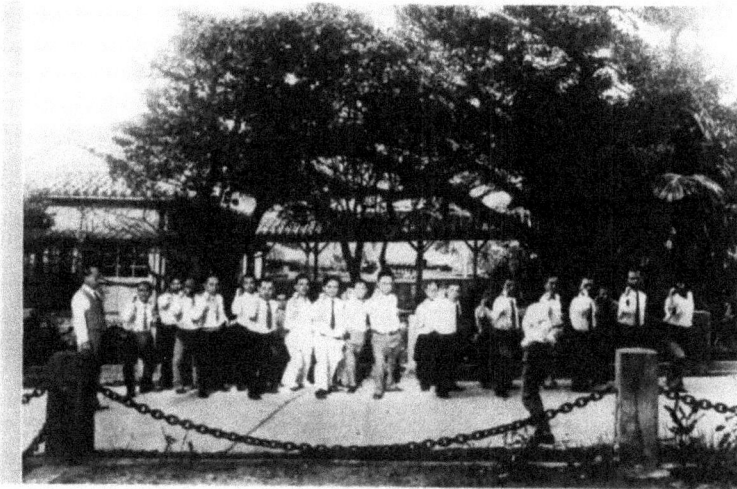

Court employees practicing Karate 1938
Employees of the Naha Courthouse training Karatedo for an hour after lunch under the shade of a tree. On the left is head judge Hirayama and on the right with his back facing the camera is instructor Kyoda Juhatsu (1887~1968.)

Looking back to the spring of the 11th year of Taisho, the Ministry of Education held its first ever Physical Fitness Demonstration. I travelled to Tokyo in order to introduce Karatedo. At the time almost no one had any idea what Karate was, in fact, most people had never even heard the word Karate. I also received considerate advice from his excellency Kanna Yomori, Professor Higashionna Kanjun, Kamiyama Seiryu of the Ministry of Finance, artist Kosugi Hoan, Professor Kasuya Mahiro and others. I would also like to express my thanks to the Toyama Military Academy, Imperial Army Officer's School, the Kodokan Dojo and other official offices, schools, companies and groups who invited the Shotokan dozens sometimes hundreds of times to do demonstrations and lectures. While these demonstrations were being conducted, Karate Clubs were being founded at universities and after eighteen years of dogged perseverance, we finally reached this remarkable stage that is sure to be remembered for generations. Karatedo is now recognized in the martial arts world.

Last summer, thanks to the words of Professor Torii Kuniyasu as well as the encouragement of Professors Saito Kazuo and Aikawa Takeo, the committee to plan the construction of a new Dojo suddenly crystalized. With Saigo Yoshinosuke as the president and Professor Ohama Nobumoto, who exerted a great deal of effort and had all the committee members racing about on a multitude of tasks, we soon had the Dojo on track to be completed. Today's ceremony celebrating the completion of the project is thanks to all their effort and dedication as well as the dedication of the heads of all the university Karate clubs, the Senpai and club members. This would not have been possible without your sincere dedication. I cannot express in words how thankful I am to you.

I would like to repay all the goodwill you have shown by increasing my efforts to create, through this patriotic Karatedo system, superior citizens of good character who have self-respect and health.

I offer these words in thanks to you all.

The Story of Karatedo
By Shoto
Koron **Public Discussion Magazine**
March 1941

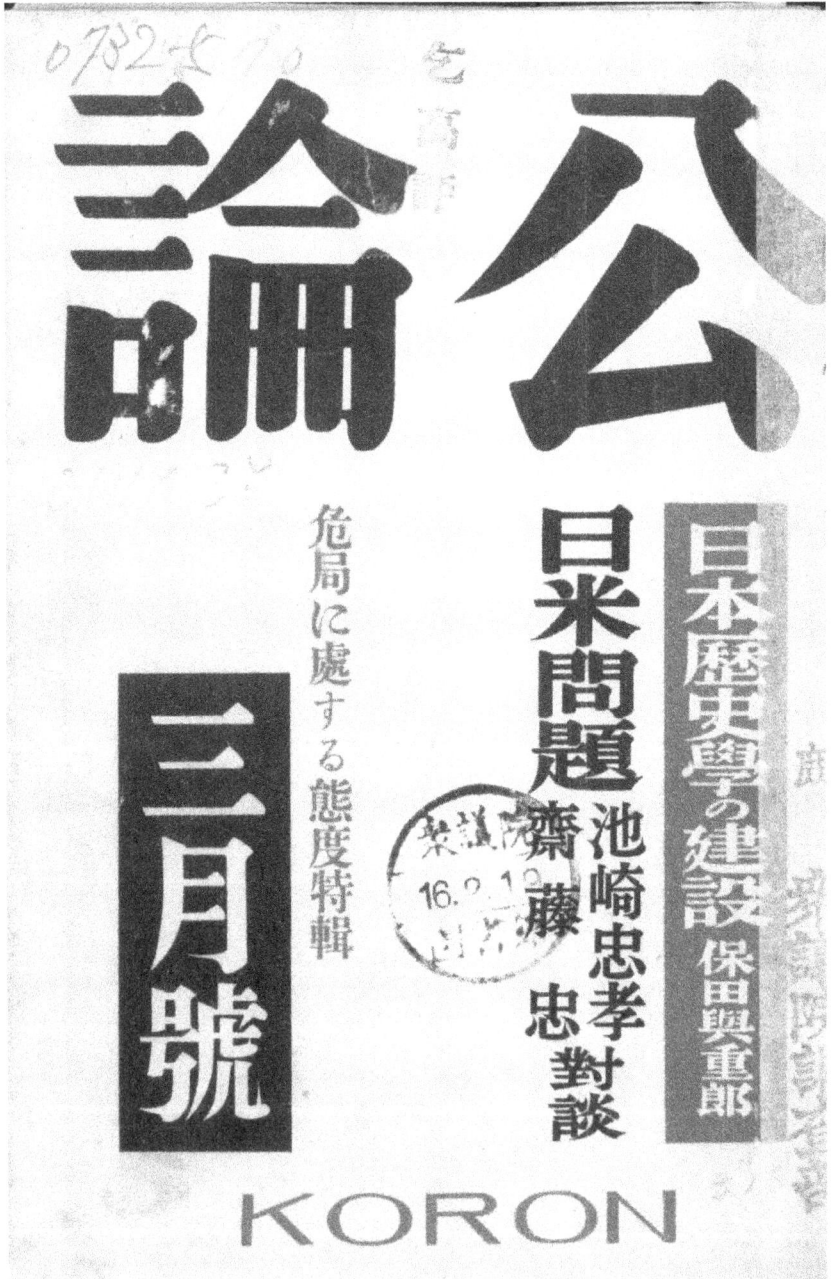

日本歴史學の建設 保田與重郎

日米問題 池崎忠孝 齋藤 忠 對談

危局に處する態度特輯

論公

三月號

KORON

The Story of Karatedo
By Shoto
1941
Introduction

There's a story about Napoleon from long ago. The French emperor was stunned to learn about a small independent country in the far east where none of the citizens had weapons. Napoleon was, of course, describing the extreme southern portion of our nation Japan, a land of Karate practitioners, which was long ago known as Ryukyu, but is nowadays known as Okinawa Prefecture.

Long Ago Karate Was Kept Hidden From Outsiders

The answer to the question, "When did Karatedo begin?" is quite difficult, because discussing Karate with outsiders was strictly forbidden. Further, this rule was so assiduously followed that no documents relating to this art have been found. Thus, it is difficult to answer that question.

It is important to note that decrees banning martial arts were issued twice in the distant past. The first was during the reign of King Sho Shin (approximately 500 years ago.)[79]

Hundreds of years ago, the main island of Okinawa was divided into the "Three Mountains." This took place around the same time as the Muromachi Era on mainland Japan. These three areas were ruled by different kings. Sho Hashi was a king of Chuzan, Middle Mountain, Ozatoaji Taromai, King of Sannan, Southern Mountain and Haneji Han'anchi was the King of Sanhoku, North of the Mountain.[80]

Each kingdom was independent and their soldiers kept their swords sharp, looking for any chance to outflank the other two. However, in the end, the king of the Middle Kingdom brought the Southern Mountain and the North of the Mountain Kingdoms under his control, and rule of Ryukyu was centralized.

---

[79] All brackets are by the author.

[80] Muromachi Era　室町時代 (1336~1573)

Central Mountain:	Sho Hashi　尚巴志	(1372~1439)
Southern Mountain:	Taromai　他魯毎	(1414~1429)
North of the Mountain:	Han'anchi　攀安知	(1376~1416)

Soon after this unification under King Sho Shin, a decree was passed ordering weapons to be surrendered to the government. At the same time academics and politically connected families were all ordered to move to the central part of the island. With that, the government by the military, became a government by legislative administration. The Marquess Sho family of today traces their lineage back to that time.

For the next two hundred years, the Samurai of Ryukyu lived in a dreamy peace until the Satusma Invasion (by Shimazu Iehisa) in the fourteenth year of Keicho, 1609 (about three hundred years ago.) Following that, another decree banning weapons was passed. At this point most historians are unified in the theory that the people of Ryukyu developed a unique *Mutekatsu Ryu*,[81] Unarmed Method of Victory School, or Karate, as a method of self-defense.

While I believe the above description is more or less accurate, I would like to make the point that I think this was more a revival of unarmed martial arts in the Ryukyu islands. One example of this can be seen during the invasion of Ryukyu by Satsuma forces. The Samurai of Satsuma were initially repelled from Naha harbor, the closest access point to Shuri Castle.

This forced the Samurai of Satsuma to change strategies and sail north to Unten Harbor and then march south towards the Ryukyu. [82]

---

[81] *Mu-te-Katsu-Ryu* 無手勝流 Empty-Handed-Victory-School. Can also refer to "Defeating your opponent without fighting."

[82] The Ryukyu warriors were aided by the fac that the port at Naha had been fortified against Wako pirates. According to Stephen Turnbull,

On two occasions, once in 1553 and again in 1556, the defenders of Naha Port had driven off wako-raids. These successes were due largely to the well-planned harbour defences that two kings had commissioned. In 1522, King Sho- Shin had built a military road between Naha and Shuri so that troops could be moved rapidly between the two key positions of the main harbour and the palace. A few years later, in 1546, King Sho- Sei had ordered the building of a small castle on each side of the harbour entrance. The two fortresses were called Yarazamori and Mie, and were linked by an iron chain that could be raised in the case of an attack.

-The Samurai Capture a King: Okinawa 1609
Stephen Turnbull

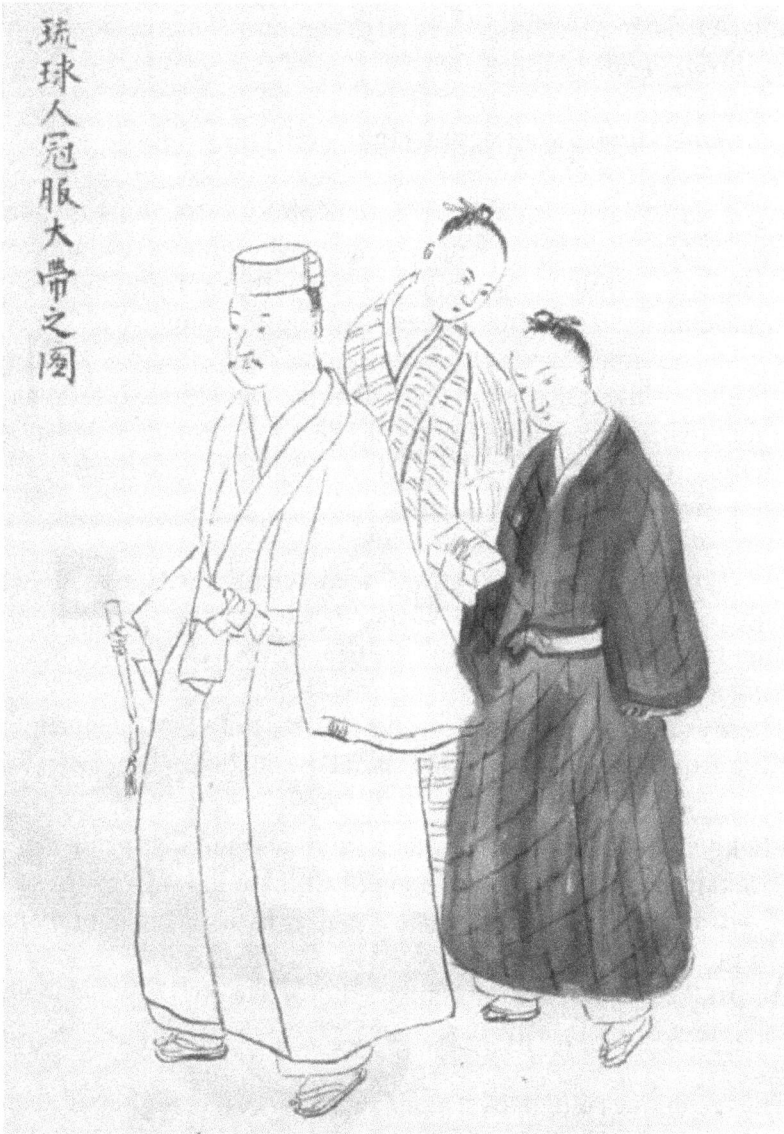

琉球人冠服大帯之図

Illustration of Ryukyu men in formal wear
Notes From the Big Island

Notes From the Big Island is a record of a 1762 incident when several Ryukyu boats bound for Kagoshima drifted ashore, a small island off Kochi Prefecture. It contains the exchanges between Confucian scholar Tobe Yoshihiro and Shiohira Pechin of Ryukyu.

Another example can be found in the story the Elder Samurai and Scholar-Official Morishiki,[83] Tobe Yoshihiro [84] wrote in his book *Notes From the Big Island*,

Kumite Jutsu Two Person Fighting Drills

Last year esteemed academic Koh Shankin (This is more of an honorific title than a name) came over with a great number of students. While his techniques used both hands, he always kept one hand guarding his breast and the technique was executed with the other hand. He also used his feet effectively and they were an integral part of the techniques he showed. Despite the fact that he appeared very weak, he accepted the challenge of a large, rough looking fellow. He was able to immediately throw the large man to the ground.

In addition, Todi Sakugawa who went to China to learn Karate/Todi and then spread what he learned throughout Ryukyu, leading to the name Todi Sakugawa becoming well-known, however looking at the dates, his travels occurred later.

There are a great many people in our prefecture that received direct training from Chinese martial artists. These include:

- Sakiyama of Izumizaki in Naha (who was the instructor to Tomi Uekata), was a disciple of Ason (a Chinese military officer.)
- Matsumura Pechin, scholar-official, was a disciple of Iwaa (a Chinese Military officer)
- Lord Azuma no Uemon Shimabukuro, student of Waishinzan (a Chinese Military officer.)

The techniques taught by a man from the An'nan region of Fuzhou, China whose ship drifted into Tomari port, were divided up as follows:

- Gusukuma of Tomari as well as Kanagusuku were taught Chinto.
- Matsumora and Oyadomari were taught Chinti.
- Yamazato was taught Jiin and Nakazato was taught Jitte

---

[83] Oshiren Shibira Pechin Morishiki 翁士璉潮平親雲上盛成
[84] Tobe Yoshihiro 戸部良熙 (1713~1796)

There is a reason that there were so many martial arts Schools around Tomari. Due to its geographic proximity, the port of Tomari is part of Naha. As it is only 1 Ri, 2.4 miles, from the seat of government in Shuri, public servants in that area were given permission to practice martial arts.

Nowadays the Dojo is Always Open

As to the question when did we start openly training Karate, I would say the answer is around 1901, the 34th year of Meiji. A certain teacher at the Upper Elementary School in Shuri began secretly teaching his students his favorite Karate techniques for an hour after classes were finished. Interestingly, when the students' physical development was being evaluated by the school doctors, they found that the students who had been training Karate were obviously healthier and had significantly better muscular growth when comparted to the students who had not trained.

This created quite a stir and at the next school principles' meeting (held at Shuri City Hall) which was attended not only by the Prefectural Head of Education Ogawa Shintaro[85] but also Itosu Sensei (my revered teacher) who, at the time, was one of the most famous Karate practitioners. [86] The instructor in question began by demonstrating how he taught Karate and the Head of Education, who was obviously very impressed, turned to Itosu Sensei and enumerated the many positive points of the demonstration. After reporting to the ministry of education, the ministry accredited the obvious physical fitness value of Karate and soon after it was publicly approved for use as part of the physical education program at the Prefectural Number One Junior High School and the Men's Teacher Training School. Thus Karatedo, which heretofore had been practiced in utter secrecy, had, through a fortunate series of events, now become an art that was taught openly.

---

[85] Ogawa Shintaro 小川鋠太郎

[86] The name Itosu is typically written with the Kanji 糸洲 However this document uses two different writings:
The first is 絲冽 and the second is 糸冽 While the Kanji 絲 is a variant of 糸 however 冽 is quite different from 洲

How Karatedo Expanded

As for when Karatedo made its way to the imperial capital, the answer is May of 1922, the 11th year of Taisho. That is when the Ministry of Education held the first National Athletic Exhibition of Japan at the site of the old Ochanomizu museum. The School Affairs Division of Okinawa Prefecture nominated me to openly introduce the uniquely refined martial art that had taken root in Okinawa. Realizing this was a great chance to introduce Karate to the center of Japanese society, I immediately agreed. I then used my calligraphy to create three large banners about Karatedo and set off from the prefectural office with a mission to explain this art to the people of Tokyo.[87]

---

[87] A 1922 Okinawa Times article describes the banners that Funakoshi Gichin took to Tokyo:

Okinawa Bujutsu To Be Introduced in the Heart of Japan
Displays for the National Athletic Exhibition have been shipped

Previously this paper reported that Funakoshi Gichin, president of the Okinawa branch of the Naobu Society has been working on the display banners for the National Athletic Exhibition held by the Ministry of Education. We have learned that as preparations are finished the banners have been sent from Okinawa prefecture on mail ship. The contents are as follows:
- One large banner describing Okinawan Bujutsu
- One medium banner describing Karate Kata
- One medium banner describing weapons and Kumite

As these three banners will serve to introduce Okinawa Bujutsu, the prefecture's top young calligrapher Shahana Unseki (1883~1975) has been tasked with the brushwork and he is sure to take this into consideration and do impeccable work.

-Okinawa Times Newspaper
April 23rd, 1922

While my plan was to return home immediately after the exhibition, I was introduced to the leading figure Kano Jigoro Sensei by Kaneshiro Saburo (an instructor at First Junior High School,)[88]who graciously invited me to extend my stay and teach some lessons. As an inexperienced practitioner, my initial response was to refuse, however I replied, "I was planning on returning home, but I can put on a demonstration." Just as I agreed to this however, it was decided that doing a demonstration for just one person would not be the best use of time so I was asked to wait for three days.

After three days all members of the upper echelons of the Kodokan were assembled along with a hundred students and teachers. As I had travelled to the capital city without a single student, I rapidly began searching for a practitioner to assist me. As it turned out, Gima Shinkin, formerly an assistant Karate instructor at the Prefectural Teachers College, [89] was currently taking classes at the Tokyo University of Commerce. I brought him along as a partner and together we demonstrated Kata and Kumite. When demonstrating the technique Kusanku, we of course did it first slowly, but we were asked to do it slowly a second time. After that we were asked detailed questions from the high-ranking members of the Kodokan (Why does your hand...?) (Why does your foot...?) and so on.

After answering questions and explaining for half an hour I was asked how long it would take to train all the Kata. I told them that to just cover the Kata would take over a year. I was honored to have them request that I teach them two or three Kata. When Imperial Japanese Army General Hishikari Takashi was principle of Toyama Military Academy and Rear Admiral Oka was the head teacher, I was asked to do a demonstration and lecture at the school.[90] Following that, they requested a week-long Karate course.

In addition, many other people and institutions, such as the Marquess Sho family, Hosokai Lawyers Association, Army Officers

---

[88] Kaneshiro Saburo   金城三郎　(1878 ~1930)
Graduate of Tokyo Teacher's College. Taught at the Okinawa prefecture teacher's college.

[89] Gima Shinkin   儀間真謹　(1896 ~ 1989)

[90] Hishikari Takashi   菱刈隆　(1871 ~ 1952)

　　Oka Takazumi   岡敬純　(1890 ~ 1973)

School, Naval Science Institute and the Nakano Military Police Academy requested lectures, demonstrations or training courses.

Upon the advice of artist Kosugi Hoan I published *Ryukyu Kenpo: Karate Jutsu*, which lead to ever greater numbers of students joining the Dojo and more schools opening. [91] And with that, I lost my chance to return to my home country.

Ages of People Training Karate

As to the question, "What is the best age to begin Karate?" my answer is, "I've taught people of every age." However, based on my experience, the ideal age to begin is around twelve or thirteen years old. That being said, I have been involved in the business of education in Naha City for over two decades and think the starting age could be lowered even further to say, students in the third or fourth year of elementary school. This is because I have seen Karate demonstrations done by fourth graders and above at city sports festivals and heard the cheers of their fathers and elder brothers, and, most importantly heard from other teachers that on days when Karate was taught at school, the school saw better attendance. I have received praise for the influence Karate lessons have had on student attendance.

Twelve and thirteen-year-olds follow commands obediently and memorize techniques quickly. Even for myself, I still vividly recall what I learned at that age.

Our art, Karate, has finally become known in the Imperial Capital as evidenced by how spectators completely filled the huge Aoyama Hall at the demonstration at two months ago.[92]

Further, last summer, I received a proposal from a motion picture company regarding making a cultural film about Karatedo. Students from the Shotokan Dojo participated in the filming of it and it was shown at over thirteen movie theaters in Tokyo. While the film was short, I believe it served as a good introduction to what Karatedo training was like in the summer.

Later, a man who appeared in that film, who shall remain unnamed, graduated from Waseda University and went to a job interview at

---

[91] Kosugi Hoan　小杉放庵（1881 ～1964）

[92] The building was finished in 1925 and could hold 2,000 spectators

Tokyo Electric. The person doing the interview recognized him from the film and commented, "Weren't you in that movie about Karate?"
"Yes, that was me."
"When doing Karate how do you strike with your fists?"
"We strike with the first two knuckles of our index finger and middle fingers. The strike should apply pressure evenly across all four of those knuckles on those two fingers."
"I would like to see exactly how these strikes are done in your art."
"Well then I'll be happy to show you a little"

So, the pair moved the chairs and tables aside in the interview room and the Karate student, who shall remain unnamed, fully committed to the demonstration by taking off his jacket and shirt before executing a Shotokan Karatedo Kata at full power.

The sound of banging and powerful Kiai shouts of *Ei!* and *Ya!* attracted the attention of the security guards to the room where an interview was ostensibly being carried out. They burst into the room thinking that the applicant had suddenly become enraged and was attacking the interviewer. At that point the interview came to an end with the result being the man was hired on the spot. "Anyone that that energetic can't help but be an asset to the company!"

The student, who shall remain unnamed, went out of his way to come to the Dojo and report the events of the day. Bowing deeply, he said, "It is all thanks to Karate!"
An extremely interesting series of events.

Karatedo is also being employed effectively by many soldiers on deployment. One such is Unit Leader Shimizu Kazuyuki who is currently in southern China. He is a ferocious practitioner, currently ranked Sandan in Shotokan Karate. Shimizu is instructing his subordinates in Karatedo. Specifically, he is teaching *Ichigeki Taiso*, Exercising the One Strike Technique, which has earned the praise of the military. This story was even reported in the Asahi newspaper.

The Ministry of Health and Welfare as also has a firm understanding of "Karatedo" and actively promotes the art through various channels. In particular, the Ministry sponsors short training courses on Karatedo at the national gymnasium several times a year.

Translator's Note

（第三種郵便物認可）　　　　九十四號

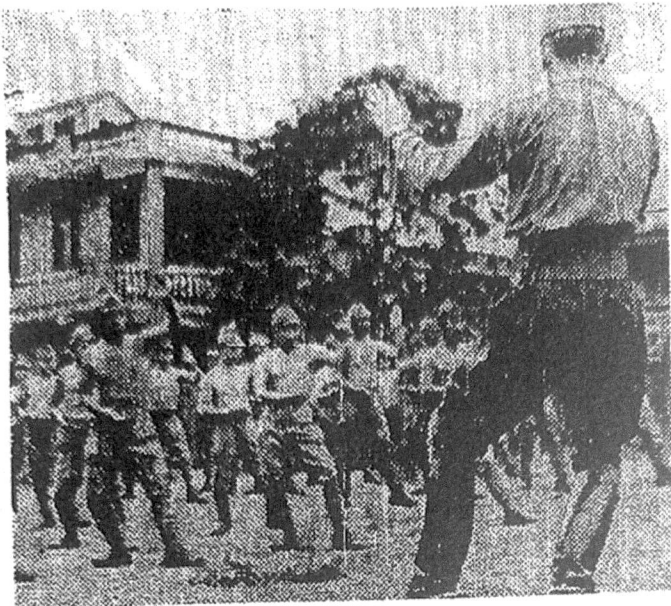

空拳敵を仆す
〝一撃體操〟
南支前線で心身鍛錬

【廣東にて堤特派員發】「一撃體操」——縣立屏東の測驗谷部隊にこんな勢ひ名のつく臨練がはやり出した〝一撃よく猛牛を斃す〟ところの空手道の型からとつたもので、手と脚を組織的に鍛錬して、さらに膽識の德と不屈の精神と勇武の氣風を鍛はうといふのだ、この「一撃體操」は六日本空手道研究會富山縣支部に籍をもつてゐる空手道二段の强者、清水和之部隊長によつて案出されたもので、仕事の餘隙上および砲聲と兵器とは絶

の違いとこの部隊が一朝有事の際、徒手空拳、身をもつて鷹を仆さといふところからこの臨練がはじめられたものであるが、いまでは各部隊にひろめられて、盛んに行はれてゐる

炎天下に午操でとび出した兵隊さん達は獵食後のひとときを割いて「えい」「おうつ」のかけ聲も勇ましく、逞しい肉體を躍動させて隨所に〝一撃よく將を斃す〟力の集團美を描き出してゐる【寫眞は一撃體操＝堤特派員撮影】

Translator's Note:

The article mentioned by Funakoshi Gichin appeared in the Asahi Newspaper on June 2nd, 1939. The translation of the article is below:

Using an Empty Hand Technique to Topple an Enemy
Exercising the One Strike Technique

Training Body and Mind on the Southern Line in China
Ichigeki Taiso, Exercising the One Strike Technique

Recently in southern China, all divisions are exercising the phenomenally named technique, "With one attack you can knock down a raging bull!" This technique originates from Karatedo, which exercises the hands and feet in a systematic method in order to forge the body. In addition, and it teaches discipline, forges an indomitable spirit as well instilling a warrior ethos. This technique is *Ichigeki Taiso*, Exercising the One Strike and originates from the Toyama Prefecture Branch of the All Japan Karatedo Research Society.

The idea was proposed by Unit Leader Shimizu Kazuyuki, a ferocious practitioner and a Nidan in Karatedo, who leads instruction, though it is beyond the scope of the usual duties of his unit, which deals with advanced weaponry. However, training in this was begun so, should the need arise, this *Tote Kuken*, Unarmed Fighting Style, will allow soldiers to topple opponents. It was originally limited to Shimizu's unit, however it has spread to other units.

Every day for an hour after lunch the soldiers stand shirtless under the blazing sun and for bravely shout *Ei! Oh!* Everywhere you look physically fit soldier are training *Ichigeki Taiso*, Exercising the One Strike Technique in perfect unison.

Photograph by Special Correspondent Tsusumu
Ichigeki Taiso, Exercising the One Strike Technique

The Origin of Karatedo

So, I'd like to go back up and explain a little bit about the origins of Karate. First of all, there's no doubt that Karate has its origins in Zen. Long ago the great reclusive sage Daruma Sensei travelled from Seichiku (present day Western India) across ten-thousand Ri[93] of high mountains and deep valleys, until he arrived in China. Where he lectured to Emperor Wu of Han.[94]

Then, in the Seiko Era,[95] (1400 years ago) he travelled Northern Wei, a land under the control of Emperor Xiaoming.[96] He settled himself at Shorinji Temple in Henan Province and began lecturing on Buddhism.

However, Daruma noticed that during his lessons, disciples would often go into a stupor and fall off their chairs. Addressing them as a whole, the Great Teacher said,

Generally speaking, the teachings of Buddha are explained in order to instruct the spirit, however your spirit and body cannot be separated from each other. From what I can see, you all are exhausted not only in mind but also in body, meaning that it is highly unlikely you will be able fully complete your training. Starting tomorrow morning, we will rise early to study the complete lessons of the Buddha.

---

[93] A "Ri" is an archaic unit of distance. In Japan, one Ri is 2.4 miles/4 kilometers. In this case 10,000 Ri refers to a vast distance, more than something specific.

[94] *There Daruma met the Emperor Wu (502-550) founder of the Liang dynasty and a devout Buddhist, who is supposed to have asked: "What is the first principle of holy teaching?" Bodhidharma's enigmatic reply, which can be translated as there is no knowing, and vast emptiness, left the emperor baffled.*

-JAANUS / Daruma 達磨

[95] Seiko 正光 (520~ 25) Japanese name for a Chinese historical era.

[96] Emperor Xiaoming 北魏孝明帝 (510~528)

From that day forward, the disciples received two methods from the great teacher: Senzui and Ekikin

Senzui is a method for purifying the spirit of toxins in order to project the wisdom from Buddha's mind (in other words, mental training.)

Ekikin is made up of two Kanji, the first means 易 Change and the second 筋 refers to strengthening the muscles of the body. Thus, the overall meaning is to train your body until it is solid and strong (in other words physical exercise.) [97]

The effect of Ekikin system is that the body develops *Kongoriki*, incredible strength, [98] and Senzui trains the spirit to have transcendental power. Thus, it is said that a practitioner that completes the training of both will have the power to move mountains and a spirit that can wrap itself around heaven and earth.[99]

Thus, Daruma is the founder of the school of martial arts at Shorinji Temple. Later, this martial art spread throughout China and has become the style of Kenpo most often seen today.

Eventually, the art made its way to Ryukyu and merged with the martial art native to Ryukyu (which was probably a martial art that resembled Kenpo.) Then, every time the previously mentioned ban on weapons was declared, the people of Ryukyu succeeded in further refining their Kenpo until the system evolved into the particular set of techniques available to us today. I would say that there is not a great difference between what we have today and that time.

---

[97] Senzui 洗髄 refers to a traditional Chinese method for training the body to discharge toxins to strengthen bones, internal organs, and muscles.

Ekikin 易筋 is a series of mental and bodily exercises to cultivate Sei (Jing or essence) and direct and refine Ki (Qi,) the internal energy of the body.

[98] Kongo 金剛 describes either a vajra (an indestructible substance) or a thunderbolt, the Buddhist symbol of the indestructible truth

[99] Ken-Kon 乾坤 heaven and earth or the whole universe.

Karatedo and Intellectual Training

Your average person thinks that learning is only something that takes place in a classroom at school, when, in fact the world outside is one big school. By simply looking, talking and listening you can gain knowledge from everything around you.

For example, as Hong Zicheng says,

Once the true way has filled your mind, there will be no place for desire to gain purchase.[100]

If your spirit is filled with the principles of justice, then intruding thoughts and distracting desires will not enter your mind.

Thinking of this in terms of a martial artist, if you have trained your body to its fullest, then there is no technique an enemy can employ that would allow his hand to reach you.

---

[100]This line is a quote from the Caigentan 菜根譚 a compilation of aphorisms eclectically combines elements from the Three teachings: Confucianism, Daoism and Buddhism. Written by Hong Zicheng 洪自誠 in 1590.

The full quote:

心不可不虚、虚則義理来居、心不可不実、実則物欲不入

*You cannot allow your mind to be filled with a multitude of overlapping thoughts and desires. The only way to allow the true way to fill your spirit is to have a mind empty of distraction. **Once the true way has filled your mind, there will be no place for desire to gain purchase.***

While walking down the road people will make way for you, a farmer plowing his field will instead hand his field over to you. If that were the case, you would have no complaints.[101]

However, if a person on the road does not make way for you, or the man farming his field does not adjust the border between his field and your, this will invariably lead to a collision. The reason for this is each person has their own desires, and this results in conflict, both interpersonal and within society as a whole.

As Sun Tzu said,

There is no doubt that man who knows himself as well as his opponent can enter a hundred battles and achieve victory every time. However, a man who understands his enemy but not his own abilities will alternate between winning a battle and losing a battle.

Obviously, it goes without saying that a man who knows neither what he is capable of or what his opponent is capable of will lose every time.

Thus Budoka, martial artists, do not dedicate themselves solely to technique, but pursue scholarly study in parallel. Failing to do this means you have no hope of becoming a true Budoka.

There is a Confusion teaching,

Not hearing a voice not seeing the shape, that describes a child sensing what the parent is thinking as an example of filial piety.

If we change the subjects of this line, it becomes a valuable lesson for martial artists.

---

[101]The countries of Gu 虞 and Zei 芮 (?~?) were in the midst of a years-long dispute about farmlands and were unable to reach an accord. They decided to consult King Wen of Zhou (1152~1050 BC) as "King Wen is a man of the highest caliber, he can tell which of us is correct."

The Kings of Gu and Zei went to King Wen's lands. They saw that the farmers were willing to shift the borders of fields in order to accommodate neighbors and peasants would step aside and allow others to pass on the road. In town, women and men walked separate from each other and you never saw old people carrying heavy goods. At court those of the warrior class were deferential to elder advisors and the elder advisors were deferential to the government.

If your mind is not there, though something may pass before your eyes, you do not see it. Though the sound reaches your ears, you hear nothing. Thus, your state of mind is the most important.

This is how Budo should look in your mind's eye. A Budoka cannot allow themselves to be held prisoner by exclusively Kata training if they wish to achieve the level described above. Failing to do so is an error. As for myself, I am part of the University System and I consider all that was mentioned above to be part of the academic realm.

Karatedo and Moral Education

The mentality of Karatedo practitioners contains the essence of Bushido. The core of this spirit is comprised of a sense of filial piety, an understanding of the importance of manners and etiquette, the necessity to be faithful to your principles, humbleness, a sense of honor, love for fellow man, diligence, endurance, persistence and an unsullied and daring spirit. All of these are what the Japanese people excel at. These virtues can be found, without exception, in all martial arts.

It is important to note that from ancient times people have said, "Karatedo practitioners do not make the first attack." This is due to the focus on mental conditioning in Karate. The recently departed "sword saint" Yamaoka Tesshu also said something exactly in line with this the philosophy, The sword that offers no aid, the sword that will not cut.[102]

However, if a situation arises and a justified response against an attempt to harm our nation, then it doesn't matter if we face a thousand men or ten thousand, do not doubt that we would immediately launch ourselves at such an enemy force.

This closely resembles the underlying thinking of Kendo. In an unavoidable situation, you will throw a punch or a kick in order to secure victory. That is why I and other Karatedo instructors pay attention to everything. And that attention is directed inward more

---

[102] Yamaoka Tesshu (1836~1888) was a fervent Kenjutsu practitioner and renowned calligrapher. He felt that the way of the sword was not a method to kill people but to bring enlightenment to the self. He is famous for his phrase *Kenzen Ichinyo* 剣禅一如 The way of the Sword and the way of Zen are one.

than out. We place emphasis on training mental fortitude, so that students develop a robust spirit focusing on training *Shin Jutsu*, mental fortitude, more than training *Gi Jutsu*, physical techniques. Rather than trying to make a grand impression, we teach students to demonstrate they can submit. Karate develops people who have soft flexibility on the outside, but a rigid strength on the inside as well as being sincere, with fortitude and vigor.

Such training will result in a modern day Budoka, martial arts practitioner, who will be of finer character and a refined physical standard. This result differs from those who slavishly follow prescribed patterns, race around trying to find new techniques, are concerned only about winning, strut down the middle of the road with their chests out and arms swinging challengingly.

If we can educate even *one* of those that mistakenly believe they are invincible and that their meager skills give them the right to pick fights, society as a whole will become healthier. It is the goal of educators, nay, it is the mission of educators to develop the people so that they may be of service to the nation.

With that in mind, my hope is to use Karate as a resource in order to further the education of the people of Japan.

Karatedo and Physical Education

If you were to look at an overview of the Karatedo exercise method, you would see that this system exercises all parts of the body. It teaches you how to move in every direction: forward, back, to the left and to the right. When training Karate, you imagine an opponent is in front of you, and attack with your hands and feet in a particular way, against a particular point on the opponent you are visualizing. It is clear that this standardized, systematic method will maximize your fighting spirit.

With that overall concept in mind, the Karatedo method also teaches how to advance, retreat, jump, move horizontally and diagonally, in addition to encouraging proper breathing. In short, this method develops all parts of the body equally and correctly in an organized fashion. Karate, it is a streamlined method designed to allow you to comprehensively develop your body in a state of harmony. This means that in a surprisingly short period of time your weak body will become strong, your circulation will improve, meaning that your complexion will be lively. This effect will be so pronounced that people will mistake you for someone else. There are innumerable cases of this.

Karatedo is a fascinating art that once students begin, they find they can't quit along the way and instead, must continue; truly a profound and mysterious art. It is probably not possible, either in spoken words or print, to describe the myriad subtleties in this art.

Further, anyone can do Karatedo. It doesn't matter if you're a man, woman, old or young. And it doesn't matter what body type you have either. Karate can be done alone or in a group, at home or at your place of work. It doesn't require any weapons and hardly any time. Karatedo is not overly complex or dangerous and the only thing you need is a desire to participate. No matter how busy a life you live, it is possible to find a way to do this training.

It can be thought of as the most effective method of rejuvenating your youth and a method for long life. You can see proof in this by the fact that, from days long past, nearly all the top practitioners in this art live to a great age. My three teachers, Itosu Sensei and Asato Sensei, Aragaki Sensei all lived well into their eighties. Matsumura Sensei was also seemingly immortal, having lived well into his nineties.

If I were to give all examples of this, I would run out of space however it is clear that Karatedo has a positive effect on health. In the end I wish for nothing less than to shout out like an orator and deliver a great speech about the physical benefits of Karatedo.

Karatedo and Kiai

The word *Kiai Jutsu*, describes using your *Seishin*, mind and spirit, to battle the mind and spirit of your opponent. In this technique you are pitting your will against your opponent's will.

Looking at this from the perspective of psychology, *Kiai Jutsu* would be described as a state where you have focused all your mental energy on a single thing, compressing every ounce of your ability until it is like a beam of light directed at a single point.

From the perspective of philosophy, this method would be described as utilizing *Kyo-Jitsu*, total freedom feints and true attacks, as well as *Do-Sei*, the unification and free use of movement and stillness.

From the perspective of Physiology, it is *Kokyu no Jutsu*, a method for regulating the breathing.

Finally, it can be simply described as *Kisaki wo Sei Suru*, stopping your opponent's attack before it even begins.

As far as examples of this technique being used, consider how Ito Ittosai used the sword technique *Musoken* to topple his opponent, or how Miyamoto Musashi used it to render Sasaki Ganryu's technique ineffective. Also, despite the fact that Araki Mataemon faced off against Yagyu Munefuyu with nothing but a white sheet of paper, Munefuyu found himself unable to cut his opponent. Other examples abound.

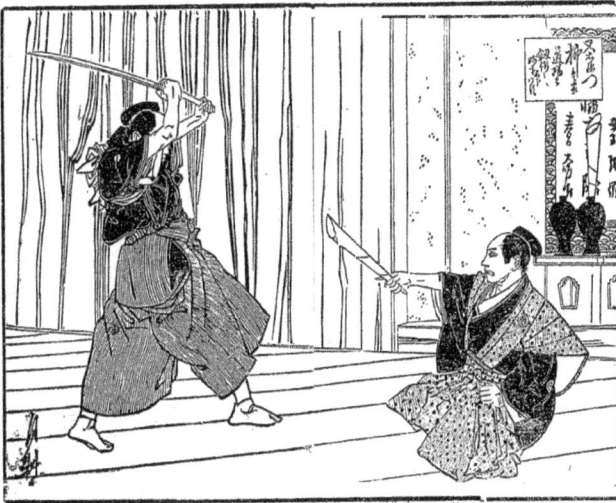

Mataemon facing off against Yagyu
From: Mataeomon (1895)

As for examples related to Karatedo, there is emperor's aide-de-camp Nakamura, who was once suspended from duty for incurred the Imperial wrath of the King of Ryukyu. Around that time a famous Karate practitioner named Uehara So-and-So formally requested a duel. Matsumura, who at this point was ready to commit Seppuku, accepted Uehara's request, figuring that by throwing himself wholeheartedly into the duel, he would end up dying anyway.

That same total commitment of body and mind to the duel must have been apparent from the intent written on his brow as Uehara, despite his standing as a Karate expert, found himself paralyzed and unable to move his hands and feet. Though he made several attempts to engage with Matsumura, in the end he was forced to remove his helmet and admit defeat.

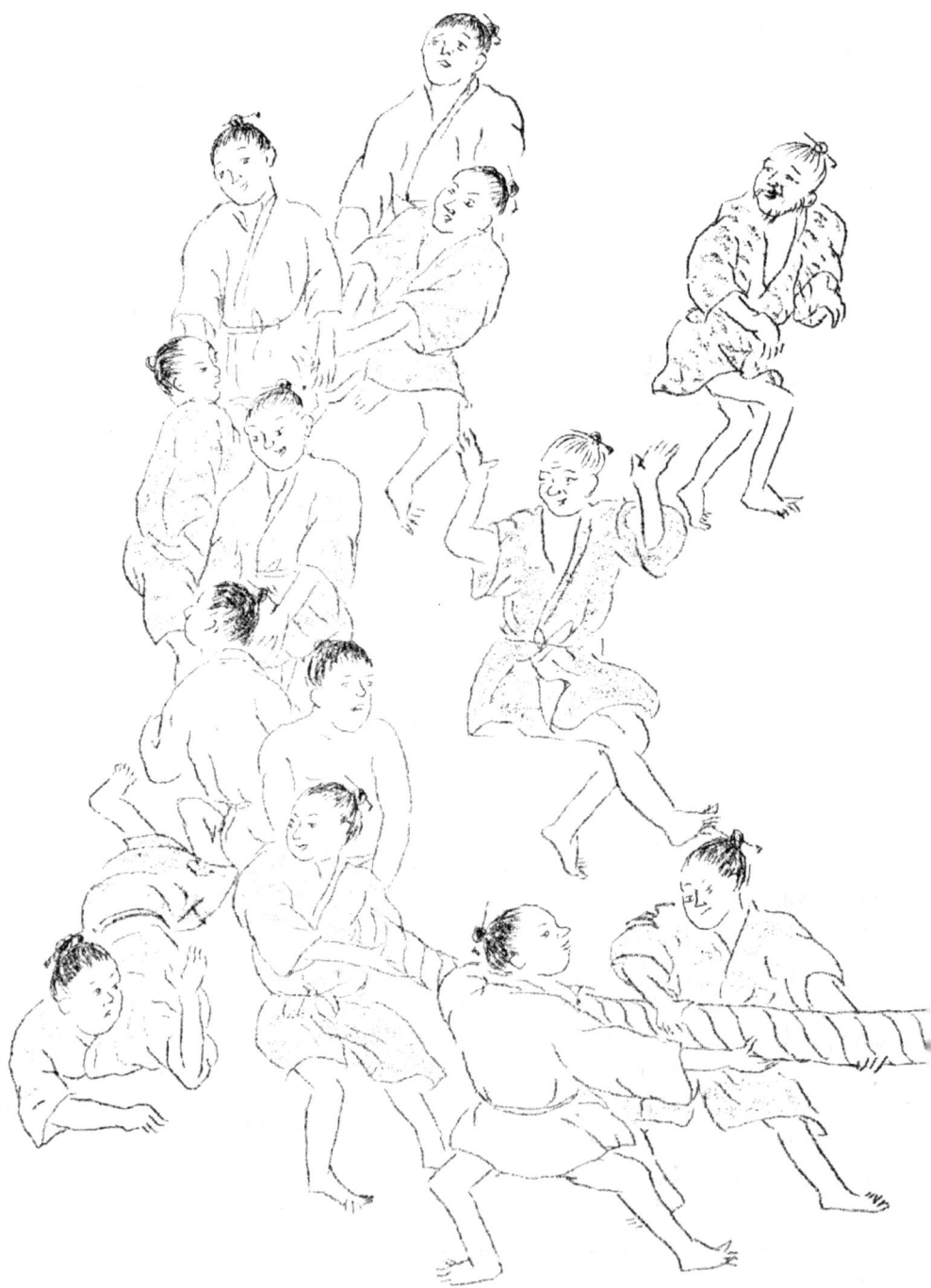

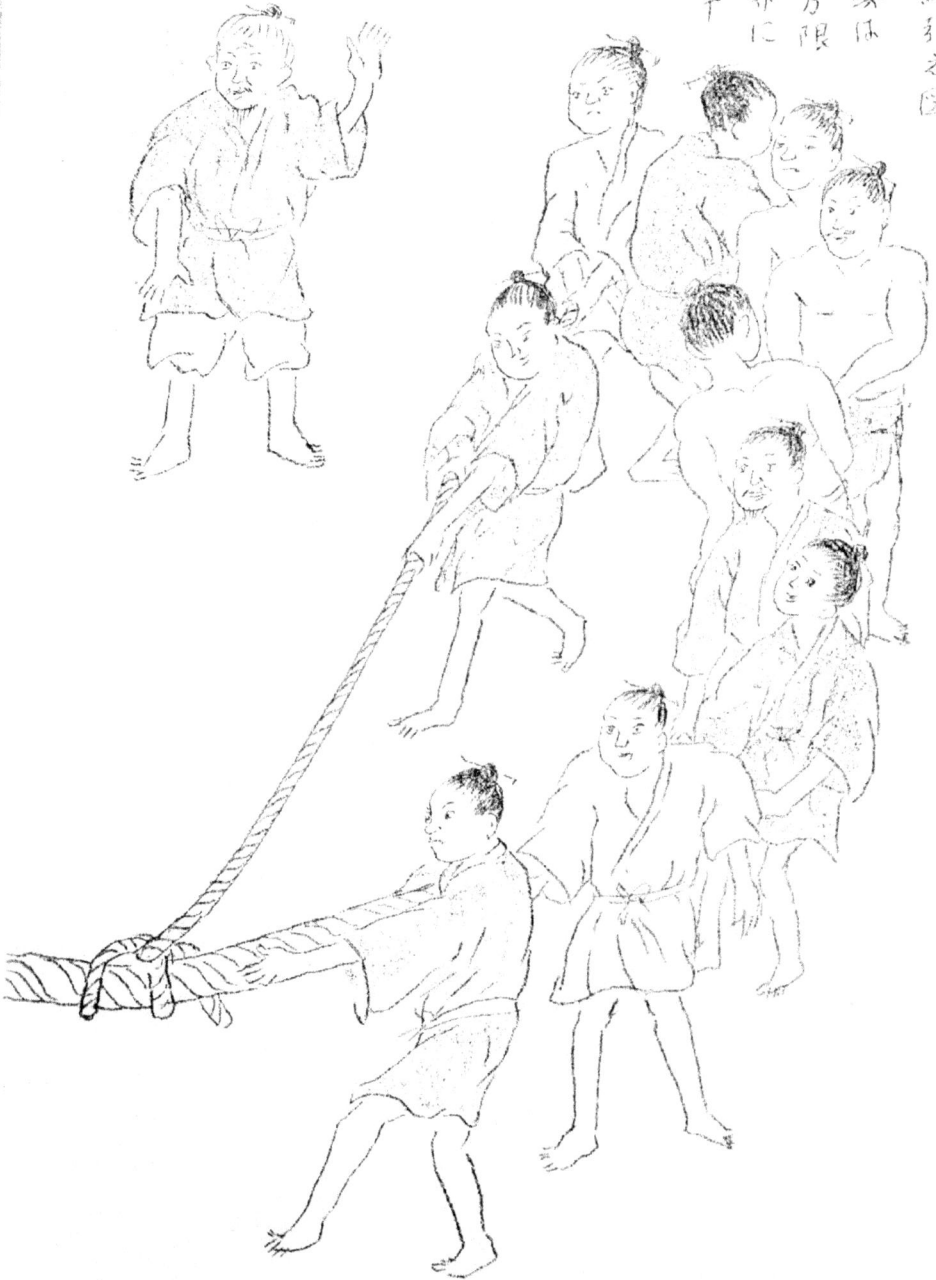

男を分て或は
村中西東方限
に分ち他界に
ひき争ふ事
なり

Also in Naha City, there was an annual tug of war event, and for some reason a great commotion had broken out that threatened to end in bloodshed. As the story goes, Higaonna Kanyu (The revered father of Higashionna Kanjun, who is currently an instructor at Tokyo Prefectural High School) appeared on the scene and scolded the entire village with such fury that through the sheer force of his personality, the attendees were all brought to submission and the event successfully concluded.[103]

In Shuri City, there is a story about a man named Ishimine So-and-So was surrounded by a group of youths while he was eating a meal. The youths were all carrying weapons. He neither became angry nor flustered but simply kept them at bay by saying, "Please wait a moment" before then finishing his food. He then stood up, took a stance and, breathing out with a sound like *Saa-Yoshi!* said, "OK then whoever's the strongest amongst you come at me!" The youths, who thought they had strength in their numbers, simply turned and left as they were overcome by his powerful force of presence.

All of these are examples of using Ki, your spirit, to control your opponent's Ki and thus can be thought of as examples of employing *Kiai Jutsu*, the art of using your force of presence to affect your opponent. A martial artist who, despite training, has not developed an understanding of this can hardly be said to be a true practitioner.

As Sun Tzu said in the *Art of War*, Winning a hundred times in a hundred battles is not the ultimate achievement, the ultimate achievement is to defeat your enemy's soldiers without even joining battle. It would be an error to think that this is not exactly what Aiki Jutsu describes.

Conclusion

So, in conclusion, Karate originated from Zen. Buddhism began in India before spreading to the Shorinji Temple in China. Shorinji temple practitioners began promulgating this art and it made its way over to Ryukyu. Shorinji Kenpo then merged with the native martial art of Ryukyu which, in turn, was refined into the art we practice today. Thus, in a broad sense, we can say that it was Japan that perfected this art.

---

[103] Illustration of a tug of war on previous pages:
Nanto Zatsuwa 南島雑話 *Tales From the Southern Isles* 1855

I would like to conclude with the current state of Karatedo in Tokyo. It has been over twenty years since I came to the capital city to spread Karatedo. From that point, I began teaching the specifics of the refined art of Karatedo and, due to the current volatile times, it is being studied by the military, the police and by people in all businesses and industries. This includes the old, the young, men and women without exception.

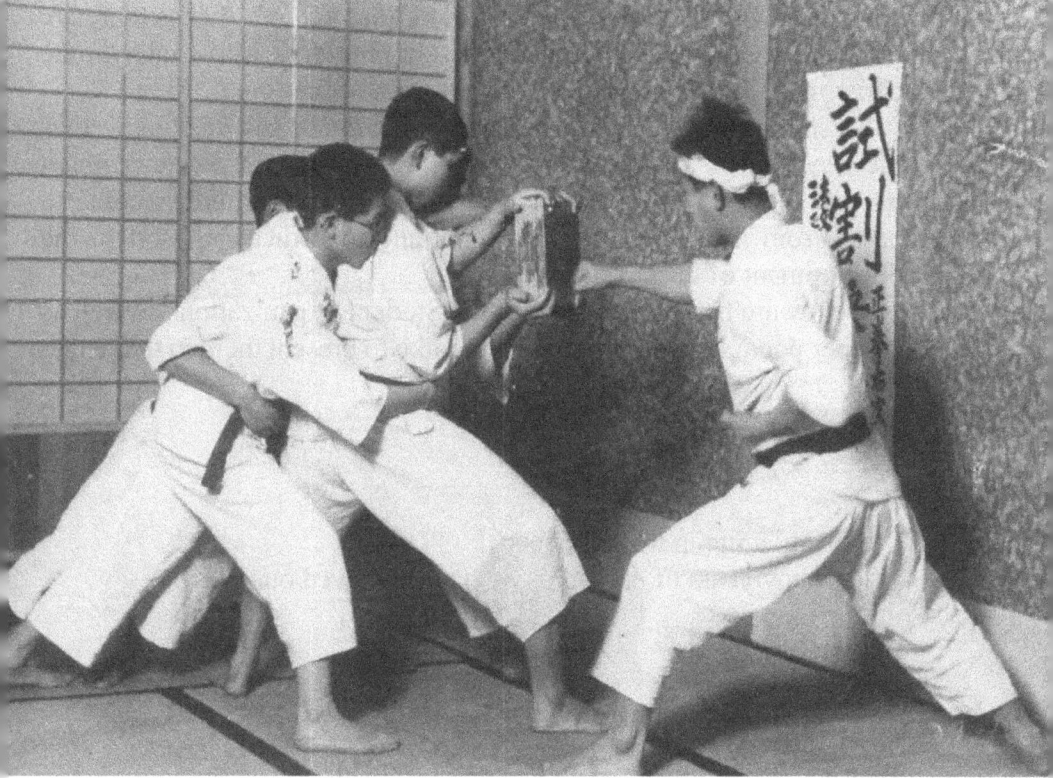

Hodai University Karate Club Tameshi Wari 1936

Various universities and specialist colleges, including many in the imperial capital, have most Karate clubs. Though founded recently, Karate clubs are seen as equivalent to the more traditional martial arts clubs at universities.[104] These Karate clubs, which were formed at schools due to the mutual interest and effort of students, resulted in

---

[104] Referring to Kendo and Judo.

more in-depth Karate research and have formed a student Karatedo organization in order to further facilitate their training

At present there are six such societies at Keio, Waseda, Takushoku, Shodai, Hodai and Ichiko universities. In addition, the Japan Medical University, Showa Medical University, Chuo University, Nichidai and others are in the process of starting clubs. There are unofficial groups at Japan Medical University and Hosei Law School, and when combined with the Shotokan Dojo at various schools means there are thirteen schools, making it seem as ubiquitous as Matsuzakaya, the department store chain. There are also private groups.

Despite this surprising expansion of Karatedo, my goal, as well as the function of this art, is to *study the literary arts while training martial arts*.[105] I am overjoyed beyond words that this has come to pass. From this point on I will continue to dedicate myself to the development of this art.

Below are two poems, one for the Student Organizations as well as another poem I have written. I would like to present them to the reader

堂々結束此連盟
辛苦多年志始成

We firmly unite in this alliance.
After many years of hardship, we have achieved our goal.

誰作中興大成業
斯心奮発誓蒼天

Who will accomplish the great task of revival?
With our hearts aflame, we swear an oath to Heaven.

---

[105] 修文錬武

Martial Arts Evening Tale : A Karate Story
By Shoto (Funakoshi Gichin)
Furusato Magazine
Part 1
July 1943

武道
夜話
空手物語（一）

松濤　述

楊先生とにんにく賣り

一

Yoh Sensei and the Garlic Salesman
Part One

The place is China. The time is long ago.

It is the day of a festival people of all ages, young and old, men and women are all wearing their finest and walking arm in arm down the street. Along both sides of the street are food stalls, shops selling clothes, trinkets, toys or firecrackers and in front of each is a salesperson calling out to customers. Suddenly people begin shouting, "It's a fight it's a fight!"

"No, it's a duel it's a martial arts duel!"

"This looks interesting why don't we go have a look!"

"No that's not what's happening. It looks like Yoh Sensei he's drunk again and looking for a fight!"

"It looks like Yoh Sensei is getting angry at some old man selling garlic…that poor old fellow he's liable to get killed!"

The whole area around the disturbance was a mass of people. Some thought it was going to be a fight, some thought it was going to be a duel, some were just drunk. The women were shrieking and trying to escape. The young men were overcome with curiosity and were pressing forward to get a better view, children were crying. All in all, the scene was total chaos.

Right in the center of the crowd was a huge man who was clearly in a fury with his chest out and arms ready, shouting about something. This was the famous Yoh Sensei. He had a wild mane of hair like a tiger and his face was shining like a Chinese red date, a redness that was enhanced by his drunkenness and anger. The source of his fury was a wobbly looking old man with white hair. This was the old white-haired fellow selling garlic and he was currently getting shoved around.

"Oh no! This is terrible, someone should say something so that old man doesn't get hurt!"

"Don't be stupid! If you get involved in this, you'll only incur the wrath of Yoh Sensei and you'll definitely regret it. The old man is up against the worst possible sort of person. Even prayers to the God's won't help"

Most of the gathered youths were cheering and shouting, clearly fascinated by the spectacle and were in high spirits since they were getting a free show. However, despite all this, the old man who was the focus of the giant drunk's attention seemed strangely unperturbed by everything. In fact, he was chuckling and said,

Well, well I'm getting a little bit sick of getting shoved around like this so I'll give you what you want and we can have a duel! You certainly are a big talker, but let's see if you can do anything except being famous for running your mouth. So, come on let's get started!

The old man coughed a couple at times and when he breathed it sounded like he was somewhat asthmatic. The crowd couldn't believe the old garlic salesman was going to take on the giant of a man, but apparently, he was serious as he started stretching his back in the everyday fashion of old men everywhere. The people in the crowd watching were dumbstruck at his apparent nonchalance. Someone said, "This is going to embed the for the old fellow. Does he know that he's going up against Yoh Sensei?!"
Another replied,
"He can't possibly know. If he knew who Yoh Sensei was, he wouldn't be saying those things"
"I have to say, I've never seen this old fellow around here before"
"I was there, when the old man realized it was Yoh Sensei! The old man said,

Ohh, he is that the guy that's drunk all year long. But he has a thousand students and he's a master teacher of Kenpo as well as sword fighting and staff fighting!

"The other day a horse broke free and was causing a ruckus, Yoh Sensei walked up and slammed his huge fist into its face and knocked it flat out!"

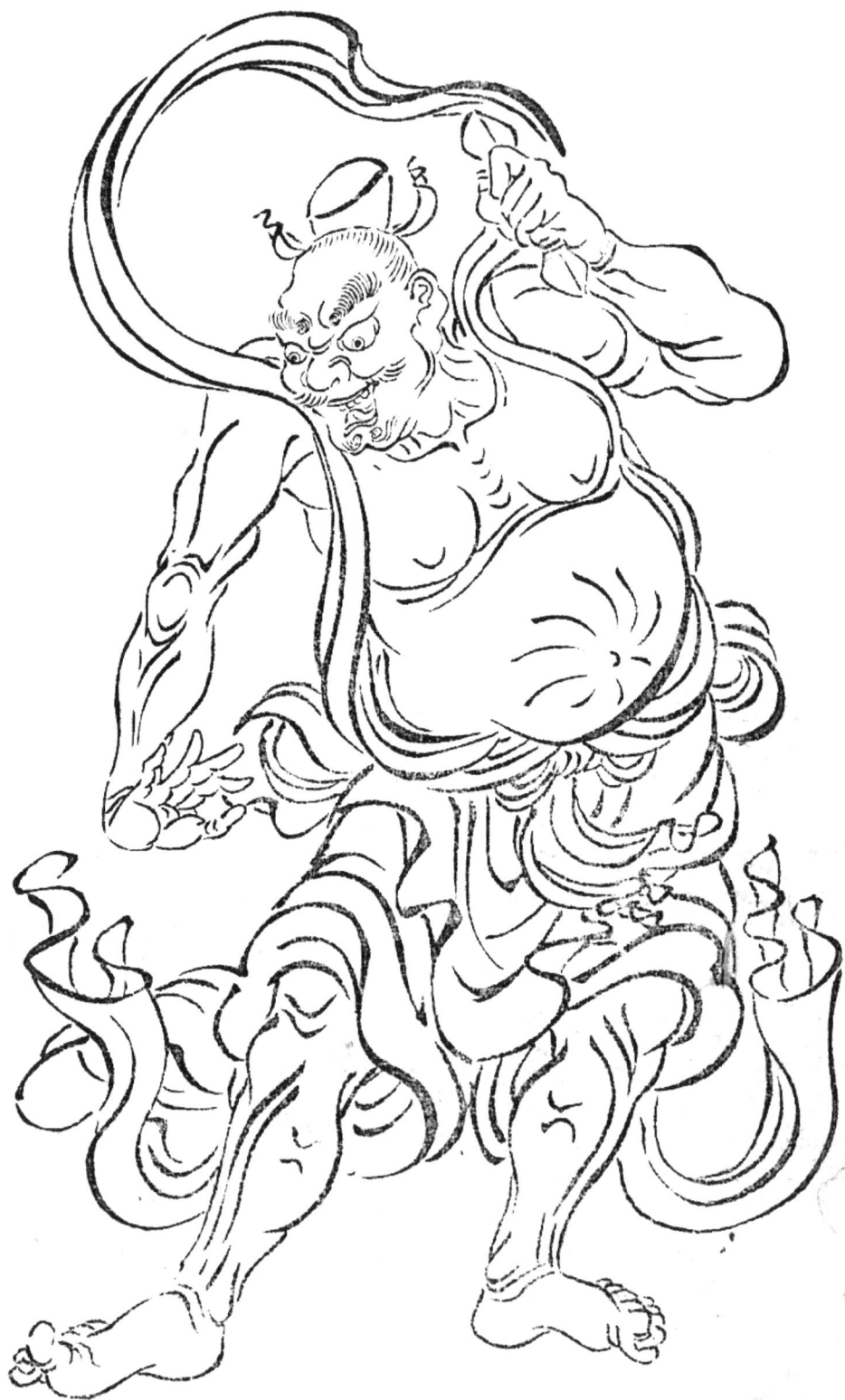

"I've seen him training with a sword that weighs two-hundred fifty pounds!"

"I've heard people say that he could stack roof tiles ten high and shatter them all with one punch from his great fist!"

While Yoh Sensei had a reputation for being a violent, angry drunk he was also a powerful man and an adept Kenpo practitioner. In the main area of the city near the castle, it was well known that no one could stand against him. However, now Yoh Sensei, a massive brute, had turned his ire upon a frail-looking old garlic seller. Curiously, the garlic seller, far from covering in terror, seemed intent on engaging the mountain of a man in a duel. Everyone watching the scene was astounded and even Yoh Sensei seemed somewhat taken aback, however in the end the old man's impertinence just made him even angrier.

"You foolish old man! At first, I thought I would leave you alive, but that time has passed! So then, if you are ready to go, I suppose I'll have to start things off...*Eiii! Ya!*"

To those about, Yoh Sensei's attack was so powerful it looked like Nio, a guardian god of Buddhism, had gone insane.[106] Yoh Sensei's fist rocketed towards the old man's head with frightening speed. All the people watching gasped, sure in the next moment that they were going to see the old garlic seller's shattered head lying on the ground, however, instead, they gasped in bewilderment. The old man was not laid out on the ground where they expected, instead the old man had simply slipped aside and allowed Yoh Sensei's ferocious attack to pass him buy. The momentum of his swing caused Yoh Sensei's fist to drive directly into a pile of sand, which sprayed all over his face. As for the old man, he now stood swaying slightly off to one side.

---

[106] Previous page:
Nio guardian (1794) by Kitao Masayoshi 北尾蕙斎 (1764~1824)

Yoh Sensei and the Garlic Salesman
Part Two

"What!"[107]

The people watching all exclaimed in unison. Seeing that his first attack had failed Yoh Sensei scrambled to his feet, quickly gathered himself and launched another attack this time aiming to strike the old man right in the stomach.

Thud!

Hearing that sounds everyone realized that Yoh Sensei's attack had struck home. The gathered crowd gasped and shut their eyes. They were sure the attack had knocked the old man flat and no one wanted to see him rolling around on the ground vomiting up blood. However, as it turned out, that was not the case. The old man who had just been struck in the stomach remained standing with a placid expression on his face. There was absolutely no change in his demeanor and he was still the same frail, rumpled looking old man with a smirk on his face.

As for Yoh Sensei's fist, it was still stuck to the old man's stomach and Yoh Sensei was coming to the realization that he could neither press forward nor could he pull his hand back. His fist was trapped, meaning all his flapping around trying to free himself, just made him look like a dragonfly. The eyes of everyone watching went wide at the curious end to the duel.

Looking carefully at the scene, it turns out that Yoh Sensei's humongous fist, which was the size of a melon, was trapped in the wrinkles of the old man's belly and he couldn't yank it free. The giant man whose physical power was second to none, was now pouring with sweat as he tried first to push and then pull, but nothing worked and he couldn't move. Turning bright red, he tried to scramble with his feet but nothing seemed to help. Thus, it came to pass that the powerful Yoh Sensei began to gasp with panic before finally being overcome with fear and sinking to his knees in front of the old garlic salesman. He then Kowtowed with his arm still trapped.[108]

---

[107] Funakoshi Gichin uses the English word "What" here.

[108] *Sanpai Kyuhai* 三拝九拝 Kneeling three times and knocking your head on the ground nine times. The historic Kowtow is to kneel, knock your head on the ground three times then stand. Repeat the process twice more.

"Since I have seen you for who you are. Up until now I was blinded by tunnel vision and did not realize you were a great teacher! I have completely humiliated myself and I vowed to reflect on this! Please take pity on me and forgive my lapse of judgment!"

The old garlic seller looked down at Yoh Sensei with a broad grin on his face.

So you finally realize the truth, I suppose that is enough. You've certainly spent a lot of time bragging about yourself, but remember the world is a wide-open place so it's best to keep your mouth under control!

With that, he released the power in his stomach and Yoh Sensei's hand was suddenly free. No longer trapped, the giant man fell back onto his butt. However, the old man didn't even glance at him again and instead turned, picked up his boxes of garlic, threw them on his shoulder and went tottering off, wheezing and coughing like he had asthma.

Overly Favoring Someone to their Detriment [109]
Part One

A lot of martial arts stories, especially the ones from long ago seemed to overdo it. Part of the reason is because the person telling the story is trying to show off, but also a little bit of exaggeration is more interesting to the listener. Thus, stories tend to be twisted over time and end up more like myths than actual accounts. The previous story about Yoh Sensei and the old garlic salesman is clearly one of those.

In Martial arts stories, you do want to hear things that are extraordinary and sublime, however if the speaker goes overboard you end up with stories like the previous one.

In Karate, there are a lot of rumors that spring up regarding the fact that practitioners are known to possess enormous power. While some of the stories are understandable if you use common sense, others, despite clearly deviating from reality, are presented as something the speaker himself has experienced. If a small child were to believe such tales that would be one thing, but I am constantly astounded that people well into adulthood seem unable to separate fact from fiction.

---

[109] 贔屓の引き倒し doing someone a disservice by showing too much partiality

There is a book that describes the power of the Karate strike Nukite that goes as follows,

> There is a secret technique called *Nukite*, Piercing Hand, that involves slamming all five fingers into your opponent's side so that the tips of your fingers pierced through the skin into the flesh. You then seize a rib and yank it out. The training you must do to achieve this strike is no easy feat. First fill a bucket with two or three *Kin*, 2.5~4 pounds, of beans.[110] Then practice slamming your hand into the bucket with your fingertips joined together.
>
> At first, the skin on your fingertips will split and bleed from repeating this first thousands of times, then tens of thousands of times a day, however as your fingers harden, your hands will begin to change shape. After even more repetition that level of training will become mundane. Having graduated to the next step, you then fill the bucket up with sand instead of beans. After switching from beans to sand, you will find it is harder for your hand to pierce through, however with days and months of practice you will eventually be able to stab your fingertips down through the sand to the bottom of the bucket.
>
> After graduating from sand, you then switch first to gravel and then to small stones, before finally training on a bucket full of lead shot. Having completed this training, you will be able to slam your fingers through a board, break rocks and easily punch through a horse's stomach.

A person unfamiliar with the subject will believe this to be true. *Karate is an amazing art! They can pierce right through a person's stomach and grab a rib and yank it out! Karate is a fearful art!* And so on.

Average people ask the most unbelievable questions,

"So, you are a Karate practitioner? That means you can smash rocks with your fists and stab a hole in a person's stomach with your finger?" Any practitioner asked such a question can only smile grimy and answer, "I can't do any parlor tricks like that."

---

[110] *Kin* 斤 is an archaic unit of weight. 1 Kin is 1.3 pounds/600 grams.

At least that is how they should answer if they don't want to exacerbate the situation. Unfortunately, some tend sidestep the question and answer along the lines of,
"Ha, ha, well, I can't say that is something I never do."

When practitioners respond like this, it invariably leads to troublesome explanations later. Invariably the Karate Sensei most likely to make such exaggerated statements is also one gifted with words so those listening are completely taken in by the speaker's riveting way of telling a story. While the speaker's true intention may be to gilt the name of Karate, in the end the result of his exaggerations is to smear the name with Miso paste.

While this is not exactly the same as the story with Yoh Sensei, when speaking glibly about Karate, no matter how difficult or strange the technique may be, it comes out as sounding like a trivial thing anyone can do. Long ago there may well have been some practitioners that could perform those feats, however, to the best of my knowledge, there is not a single Karate Sensei alive today who can do those things.

Overly Favoring Someone to their Detriment
Part Two

There are Karate Sensei that say things that seem to serve only to blow smoke in the eyes of the uninitiated.
"Grip strength is the most important thing in Karate. Thus, in order to train grip strength, we find jars with very small ridges around the tops, just enough for the fingers to grip. We then pack them all the way to the top with sand and hold one in each hand and swing them around. A person who has done sufficient grip training can seize an opponent's hand or leg and rip the flesh from the bones."

While parts of this story are true, the bit about rending flesh into a thousand pieces is an exaggeration. Human flesh is hardly the same thing as pulling Mochi, pounded rice cakes, into shreds.

There was once an iron factory worker who came to the Dojo. He said that since he was constantly using just the fingers of his right hand to pull iron plates out of the machine that made a hundred kilometers of the plate a day.

Since he had spent long hours training the fingers of that hand, his fingers had become spectacularly powerful and he felt that, while it was unlikely he could rip a man's rib out, it seemed likely he could rip a chunk of a man's flesh from his body. Since the man seemed so serious, I decided to give him a chance and took my shirt off.

"Why don't you try and yank some flesh from my side!"

The man was somewhat taken aback that his boastful proposal had been accepted, however he couldn't back down now. He grabbed my side as hard as he could but, as I had put power in my muscles, all parts of my body became rigid. This meant that, much to the iron worker's chagrin, he had trouble even finding something to grip. It would be one thing if he was simply some uninformed person, but the fact that this self-styled Karate master went out of his way to boldly enter my Dojo and attempt to teach us the secret technique of how to strip the flesh of a person into a thousand pieces, simply beggar's belief. We had him start his demonstration right away, but there didn't seem to be anything to his technique. All that happened was I got a bit of a bruise. In the end we all had a laugh as despite the fact that the iron worker was attempting to "rend flesh into a thousand pieces" the result was barely leaving a mark.

It seems there is a limit to how far your grip strength can be increased. Of course there were people who were blessed with fantastic strength. For example, people that could hand from the roof beams of houses and go hand over hand all the way around the building. That being said, you should consider how houses are built in Okinawa.

Martial Arts Evening Tale : A Karate Story
By Shoto (Funakoshi Gichin)
Furusato Magazine
Part 2
December 1943

武道夜話

空手物語 (一)

松濤 述

空手の淵源

The Origin of Karate
Part One

It is said that Karate originated from Chinese Kenpo. As there is also a theory that Chin Genpin is the one who brought Jujutsu to Japan, I will also include the theory about the origins of Karate.[111]

Obviously in human society, if a war occurs, it implies that there was some type of fighting art already in existence. Even if in a given society, bronze or stone weapons have not yet been invented, surely some form of unarmed combat existed. It would be childish to try and describe that as a wholly formed art, however there were surely people that were skilled at fighting and those that were bad at fighting. And it follows that, perhaps, some people realized who was good at fighting and began to copy that person's way. Thus, if you want to find the origins of Karate, that is how far back upstream you have to search.

During the reign of Emperor Suiun (69BC~70AD,) there was a man of unparalleled strength and bravery who lived in Taima village in Yamato Domain. He could straighten out iron hooks with his bare hands and twist a bull's horns until they broke off.

In particular, he could apply his legs deftly, even going so far as to taking the nickname Kehaya, Fast Kick. He would often comment to people,

"If there is any man in the world who would like to try his power against me, I will fight him to the death anytime and anyplace."

Such bragging even reached the ear of the emperor who asked his advisor,

"Kehaya makes no effort to disguise the fact that he is the greatest Sumo wrestler in the land, is there truly no man who can best him?"

"In Izumo Domain there is a man named Nomi no Sukune. He was born with an incredible amount of strength. I believe that Sukune could defeat Kehaya."

---

[111] Chin Genpin 陳元贇 (1587~1671) was a Shaolin practitioner who travelled to Japan and introduced techniques to Samurai that were incorporated into Jujutsu.

With that, the Emperor ordered that both men be summoned and ordered to duel. The moment the fight began, both men leapt forward. Sukune turned his opponent's special attack against him. Sukune's first kick cracked Kesoku's ribs, and as Kesoku dropped back in pain, Sukune followed up by stomping down on his pelvis, shattering it. Even the great Kesoku couldn't take such a beating and he died. Apparently, this duel was a spectacular one rivalling any of the Samurai duels in the warring states period.

The emperor praised Sukune's bravery and granted him the Taima region lands in Yamato Domain. After that, Sukune remained in Yamato Domain and continued to serve the Emperor. Later, he was revered as the founder of Hajibe potters, as he was the one who proposed abandoning the practice of sacrificing people to accompany royal burials and use clay Haniwa figures instead. Clearly a man of profound wisdom and strength.

Later, Nomi no Sukune would be hailed as the god of Sumo. However, as he was able to take down Kehaya, a man famed for his nimble legs and feet, with a single kick, it seems the great historical martial art he is responsible for founding is not at all like Sumo or even like Judo, quite mysteriously it seems to look almost exactly like the leg techniques found in our Karate.

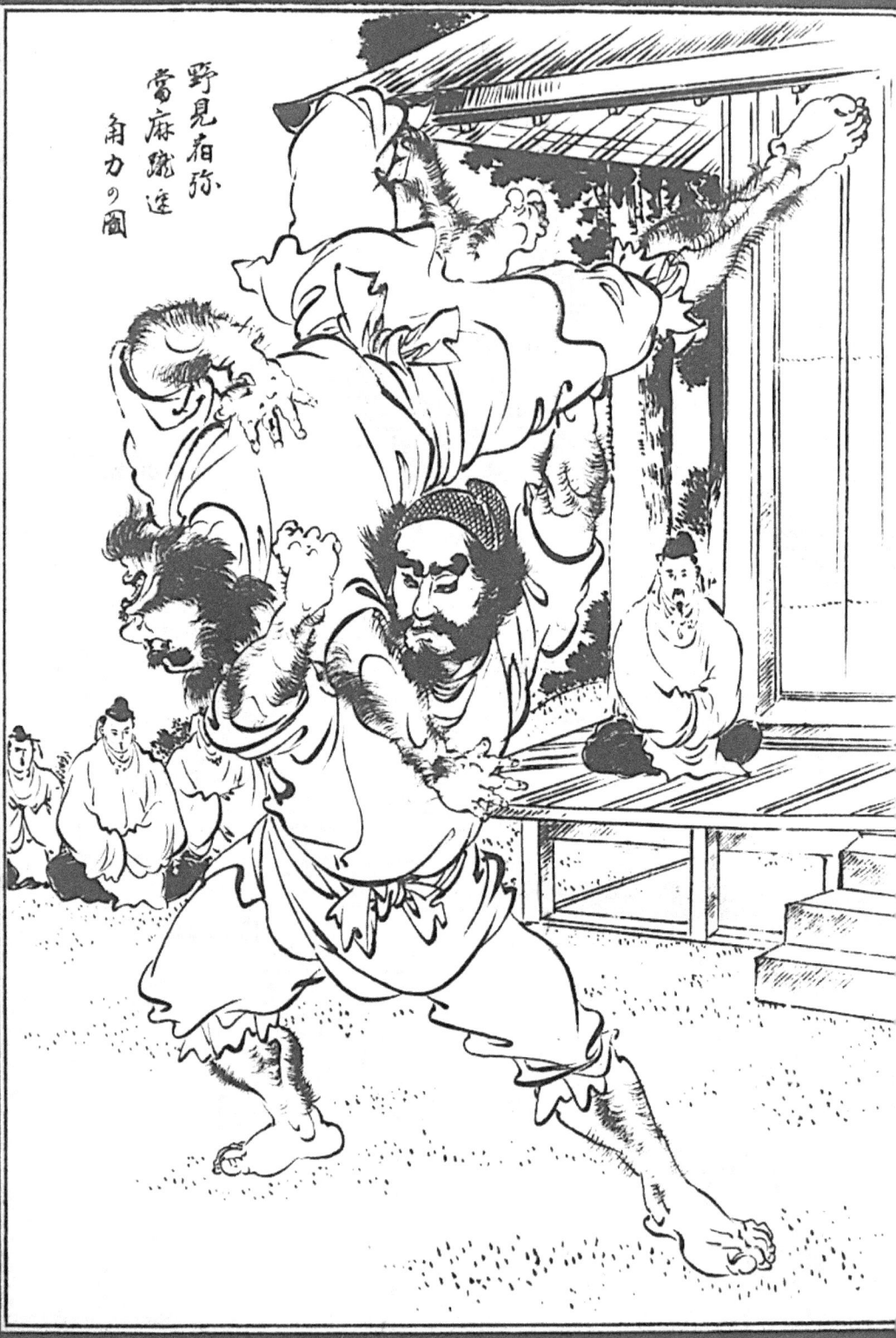

野見宿弥
當麻蹴速
角力の圖

Translator's Note:

Funakoshi Sensei is paraphrasing *Nihongi*, The Chronicles of Japan, a history book finished in 720 AD. This book was written in Chinese. The illustration on the previous page of the duel between Sukune and Kehaya is from The Chronicle of Japanese Sumo 本朝相撲沿革 by Matsui Isojiro 松井磯次郎 and was published in 1922. This is a translation of the relevant section from The Chronicles of Japan.

7th year, Autumn, 7th month, 7th day.

The courtiers represented to the Emperor as follows,

"In the village of Taima there is a valiant man called Kehaya of Taima. He is of great bodily strength, so that he can break horns and straighten out hooks. He is always saying to the people, *You may search the four quarters, but where is there one to compare with me in strength? O that I could meet with a man of might, with whom to have a trial of strength, regardless of life or death.*

The Emperor, hearing this, proclaimed to his ministers, saying: *We hear that Kehaya of Taima is the champion of the Empire. Might there be any one to compare with him?*

One of the ministers came forward and said: *Thy servant hears that in the Land of Izumo there is a valiant man named Nomi no Sukune. It is desirable that thou shouldst send for him, by way of trial, and match him with Kehaya.*

That same day the Emperor sent Nagaochi, the ancestor of the Atahe of Yamato, to summon Nomi no Sukune. Thereupon Nomi no Sukune came from Izumo, and straightway he and Taima no Kehaya were made to wrestle together. The two men stood opposite to one another. Each raised his foot and kicked at the other, when Nomi no Sukune broke with a kick the ribs of Kehaya and also kicked and broke his loins and thus killed him. Therefore, the land of Taima no Kehaya was seized, and was all given to Nomi no Sukune. This was the cause why there is in that village a place called Koshi-ore-da, i.e. The Field of the Broken Loins.

Nomi no Sukune remained and served the Emperor.

- Chronicles of Japan
William George Aston
1896

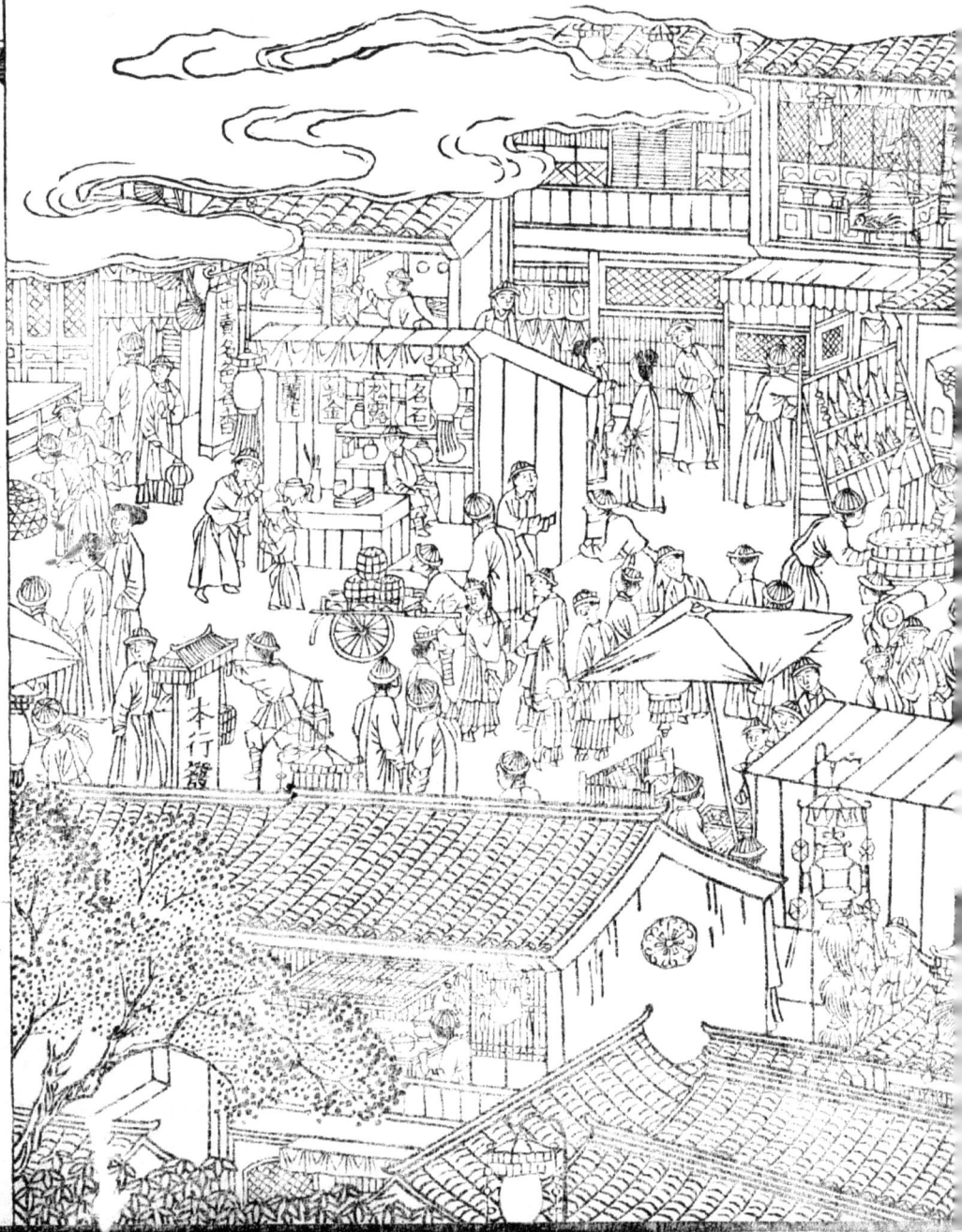

琉球の國交易繁栄の圖

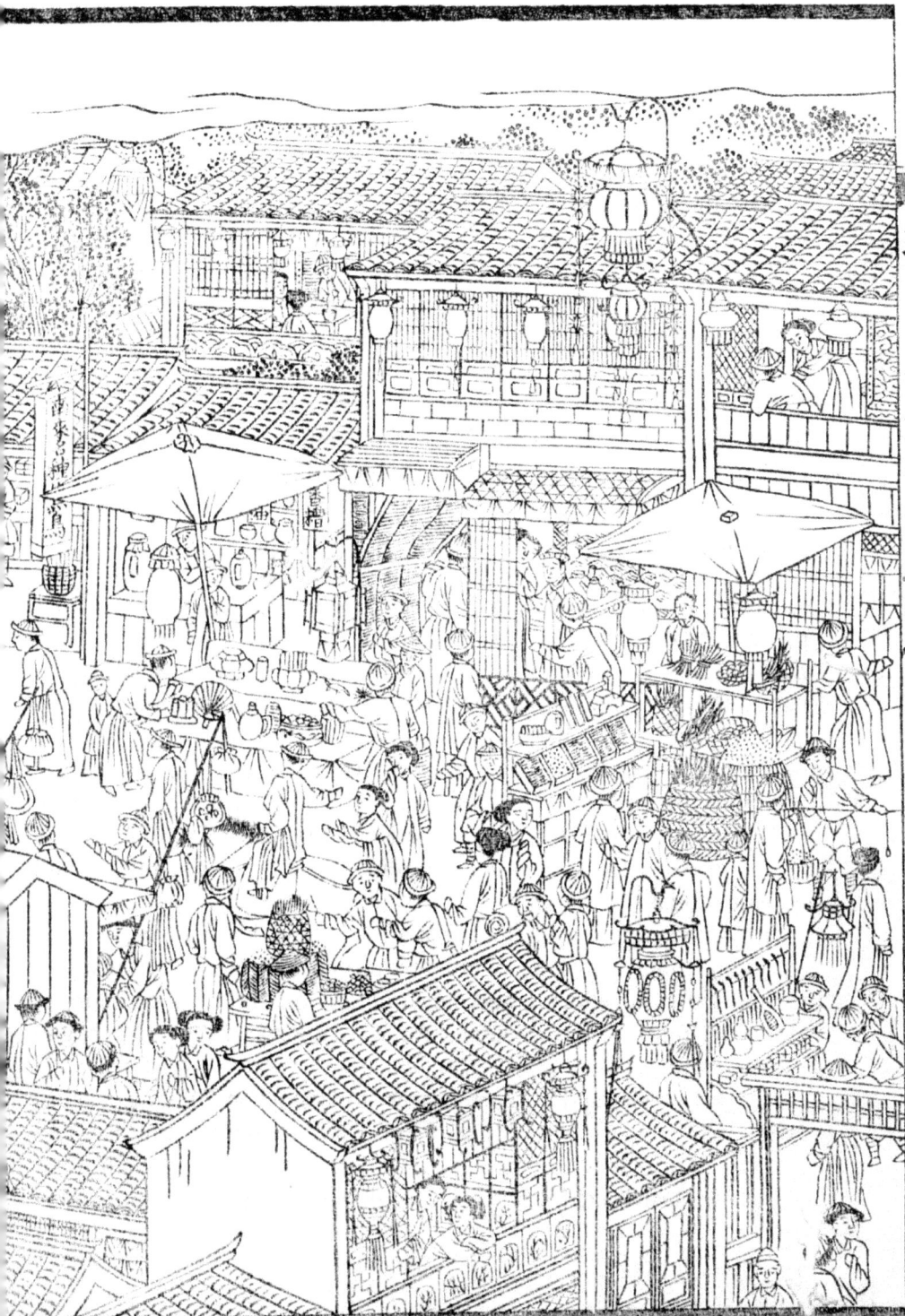

The Origin of Karate
Part Two

In short, in the initial stages of its development, the martial art of a given country is going to differ from that of other countries at that same stage in their evolution, as it will reflect the nature of the people that develop it.

The duel between Kehaya and Nomi no Sukune took place in the seventh month of the seventh year Emperor Suiun's reign. Thus, historically speaking, it took place in the Imperial Year 638, or 23BC, more than two thousand years ago.

Chinese Kenpo, which is said to have been founded by Daruma of India. He travelled to meet the Emperor Wu (502~550) and lectured to him before settling at the Shorinji temple and teaching Buddhism. As this was in the Seiko era, 520~525AD, in Northern Wei, this is about six hundred years after Sukune's time. During his time at the Shorinji temple, Daruma taught the monks methods to forge not only their minds but also their bodies. The methods he taught were called Senzui and Ekikin and this was considered to be the beginning of Shorinji Kenpo.

Even today the Kenpo taught in China and Manchu Domain is mostly derived directly from Shorinji Kenpo…or so it is said. Other names for this art are *Kokujutsu*, National Art, *Shorin-Ken*, Shorin Fist, *Daruma Ken*, Daruma's Fist, and others, however despite the different names they are broadly similar and only vary in the details

The fact that Chinese Kenpo had a big influence on the development of Okinawan Karate is clearly due to the geographic proximity of the two nations. While such techniques are not used in the Shotokan, it is a fact that some Karate practitioners in Okinawa train Chinese Kenpo Kata that are remarkably similar to ones found in China today.

Thus, to suddenly conclude that all Karate is derived from what is taught in China is an error of colossal proportions as for the most part it was either developed and nurtured in, or purely a creation of Okinawa. Further, the research into systemizing this art only began extremely recently.

The Karate being done currently at universities in Tokyo as well as vocational schools, the Ministry of Welfare demonstrations and lectures is primarily this newer method of teaching Karate. In other words, the systemized Karatedo. I would like to make it clear that this is a new version of Karate that does not resemble the Karate of the past. [112]

The secret martial arts of Karate.
Part One

There are no historical documents or books related to Karate. Thus, we cannot say who founded it, the lineage from that person until now or any other related information. The little that we do know is from orally transmitted stories and those orally transmitted stories themselves are ambiguous and trying to understand them is like grasping at clouds. The reason for this is because as late as the era when I and my fellows were training Karate as young men, the art was not done publicly. We were admonished again and again to keep secret the training we did as well as any kata we learned. The Karate Dojo that you see nowadays simply did not exist in the past, thus Karate teachers at that time we're not teachers by trade rather they had another means of earning a living.

Men such as Matsumura who was a famous Karate practitioner served as a martial arts instructor to the King of Ryukyu, but Uehara, the man who challenged him was an engraver. Recent men who are famous Karate practitioners such as Asato Sensei, who took special care to instruct me, was known as Tonochi, a Ryukyu word that refers to the head of a minor domain. He was my teacher for ten years and he taught me Heian and Tekki as well as other techniques. Ito Sensei, who served as an official scribe to the King of Ryukyu.[113] As there was no one that worked as a Karatedo instructor as their main profession, there wasn't a lot of emphasis placed on traditional aspects of the art. They taught people as a hobby. The people that took Karate lessons did so because they enjoyed it. That is why at the time I trained

---

[112] Previous pages:
Scene of a busy street market in the Ryuku Kingdom before the Satsuma Invasion
From:
Illustrated Record of the Ryukyu Campaign 絵本豊臣琉球軍記
1836

[113] *Goyuhitsu* 御祐筆 Honored Scribe to the Right. This was more than just writing what the King said, scribes would also draft documents for public dispersal and maintain political records.

with Asato Sensei, despite him being a generational talent, had only me as a Karate Student. Even when I was training with Asato Sensei, there were almost no students. Nowadays, even the smallest and poorest local Dojo has more students than what he had. The tradition of keeping all information about training secret was a generally practiced tradition until recently.

The secret martial arts of Karate
Part Two

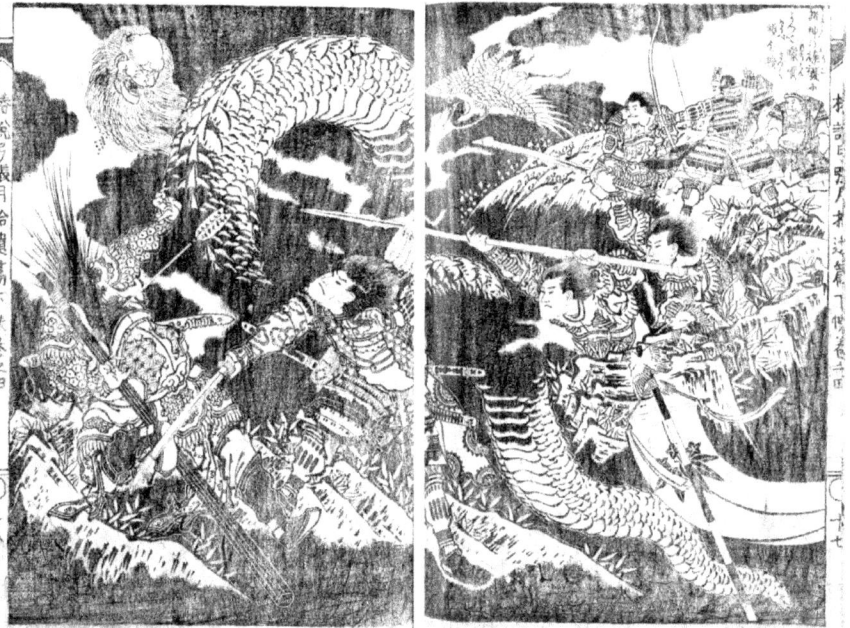

Crescent Moon: The Adventures of Tametomo
by Katsushika Hokusai 1807
A dramatic retelling of how Minamoto no Tametomo came to Ryukyu

The expansion and development of Karate in Ryukyu happened due to two government decrees banning weapons. Around five hundred years ago, during the time when the Three Mountain Kingdoms were unified by King Sho Hashi, who, historically, is said to be a descendant of Shunten, an illegitimate son of mainland royalty.[114]

Having unified the country, the king then issued a decree banning weapons, thereby making the ownership of weapons illegal. Following that, government officials and academics were all ordered to move to a central location, thereby consolidating power. Later kings of Ryukyu all descended from the Sho Family.

The next two hundred years passed like a peaceful dream until, in the fourteenth year of Keicho, when the Shimazu forces of Satsuma Domain began what is known as the "era of ferocious war in the southern seas" and Ryukyu had no choice but to join combat. When speaking of the Samurai of Satsuma domain in the warring states period, they can only be described as being unparalleled in their savagery, so much so that they even gave Toyotomi Hideyoshi a hard time.

The fierce Samurai of Satsuma turned their attention to the Ryukyu archipelago, and the Ryukyu fighters defended their land valiantly. In fact, the defenses around Naha were so strong that even the Shimazu armies couldn't break them. However, in the end, the Ryukyu forces lacked fighting experience as well as numbers and they fell for a feint by the Satsuma forces.

When the Satsuma forces suddenly sailed north and landed at Unten Port, the Ryukyu forces misread their opponent's strategy and were caught completely by surprise and defeated. With that, the entire island chain fell into the hands of the Shimazu Clan. From that time on there are no reports of average Samurai or commoners gaining fame by using weapons in the Ryukyu islands.

It seems likely that with the implementation of a ban on weapons, that the unarmed fighting technique that was already practiced in

---

[114] Sho Hashi 尚巴志 (1372 ~1439)

Shunten 舜天 （1165~1237) was the legendary first king of the Middle Mountain Kingdom. The official histories of the Ryukyu Kingdom claim that he was the son of the Samurai Minamoto no Tametomo (1139~1176?) and a local noblewoman. One version of Tametomo's story is that following the Hogen rebellion he was exiled to Oshima island. The island is south of where Tokyo is today, and he committed Seppuku, one of the earliest examples of the practice. However, another legend states Tametomo reached Ryukyu and married the sister of a local lord and had a son, Shunten.

Ryukyu began to develop quickly. At the same time, the various trade routes with China meant that Chinese style Kenpo began to appear in Ryukyu. This began to merge with the native Ryukyu martial arts, or, in some cases, be practiced on its own. Thus, before Karatedo, it is thought that Taude and Okinawa Te were established.[115]

When we were young, we often heard older folks talking about Taude and Okinawa Te, however thinking back on it, I believe when they said Taude, based on the flow of conversation they were actually referring to Kara-te, Chinese style Kenpo. On the other hand, when they said Okinawa Te it seems to me they were referring to the art that is unique to Okinawa.

The result of the official policy of banning weapons was the flourishing of a martial art that required no weapons and only used the hands and feet to protect the body. Along with that, for what reason we can't be sure, Karate practitioners kept their training and how they transmitted learning a closely guarded secret. This is what I think about that.

Entering the magnificent imperial reign of the Meiji Emperor, it was no longer necessary to conceal training, however as the tradition of secrecy had been around for hundreds of years, no one trained publicly and any transfer of knowledge was done in secret. Clearly, this concept had unconsciously taken root in people. While some of this may have been a desire to protect the *Gokui,* highest level secret techniques, from leaking out like in Kendo and other martial arts, I can't help but believe there is more to the story as secrecy was so strictly enforced and no documents remain to us.

Having unified the country, the king then issued a decree banning weapons, thereby making the ownership of weapons illegal. Following that, government officials and academics were all ordered to move to a central location, thereby consolidating power. Later kings of Ryukyu all descended from the Sho Family.

---

[115] Funakoshi Sensei writes the word Ta た u う de で

Yomiuri Newspaper
February 26th 1944

Giving the American devils an iron elbow
Girls division taking Karate training

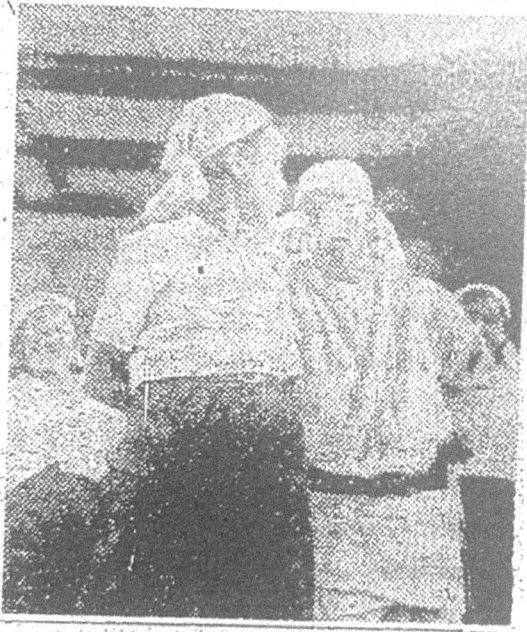

Yomiuri Newspaper
February 26 1944

Giving the American devils an iron elbow
Girls' division taking Karate training

Give the disgusting American devils a roaring blast from our iron elbows that strike like a cannon blast to the nose. Principal Yoshimura Katsumasa of Chichibu Girls High School in Saitama Prefecture has decided to start teaching Okinawan style "Karate" Kenpo to the girls.

The principal was the captain of the Karate club when he was a junior high school student in Okinawa and thus a veteran practitioner. In the fight to increase production women are stepping up to volunteer to replace the men, thus women and girls need to be instilled with a conviction that they will invariably achieve victory. Thus, the volunteer girls have become enlightened to this martial art and demonstrate their decisive martial ability as they bravely train their bodies shouting Kiai of *Ei! Ya! Ya!*

The school is planning additional training in responding to emergencies so that the girls will have the ability to respond to air raids firmly implanted this is part of our overall push for establishing Certain Victory Education.

Photograph: Girls teaching Karate to girls

Yomiuri Newspaper
September 25th 1948

Chiba prefecture holds first Karatedo public event at the education hall

Yomiuri Newspaper
September 25th 1948

Chiba prefecture holds first Karatedo public event at the education hall

The first Karatedo public demonstration will finally be held today the 25th starting at 1:00 PM at the Chiba prefectural gymnasium. This exciting event is sponsored by the prefectural gymnasium as well as supporters of Shotokan School Karate and the Yomiuri newspaper.
Practitioners from the Karate clubs at Chuo University, Waseda University, Keio University and other schools will demonstrate.
The event will begin with an explanation of the origins and development of Karatedo and Karatedo as a sport. Next will be basic techniques followed by weapons and Karate including stacking 10 roof tiles up and breaking them. In addition to breaking boards, they will also be construction belts so you can see how Karate is done.

Picture : A violent Karate kick

Karate
A Story From the Venerable Karate Authority Funakoshi Gichin
Fuji Magazine
April 1951

空手

空手の権威船越義珍翁から聞いた話である。

沖縄の首里の山川といふ紙漉き業者の部落に、石嶺という男がいた。彼がある時、農村にいついて仕事をして、帰ろうとすると、農夫が、あらぬことを言い張つて何の彼のと彼にいんねんをつけた。むつとしたが我慢をして荷を負つて帰る彼を、執拗に農夫達はこづき廻る。遂に堪忍袋を切つた彼が、右手でサツを拂いのけると、拂われた男の額が双物で切つたように、サーツと切れた。そこで「こいつ！ 双物を持つてるぞ!!」と、大聲になつた。その中、駐在所の巡査がやつて来て、石嶺は手錠をかけられて、警察につれて行かれた。警察では、いくら正常防衛を主張してもきいてくれない。ふと窓越しに庭を見ると、ヘチマの棚があるのを目に止めた石嶺が、その棚木の丸太直徑二寸、長さ二間程の自然木を一本抜いて来て貫つて、

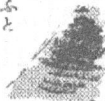

『これを手で斷ち切つて御覧に入れましよう。もし何かに使うのなら、その間尺を仰宣つて下さい。』

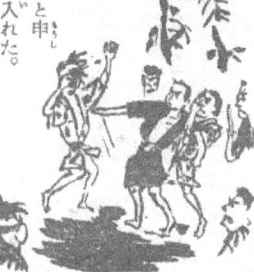

と申入れた。

ホラを吹くと思つて誰も答えるもので切つたようであつた。あつ!!と驚嘆の聲が上つたのはいうまでもない。

『えい!!』と鑿をかけると、木は下から二尺くらいの所を斜めに斷ち切つていた。まるで銳利なナ

『御希望で、どんな長さにでも――』と、警官を見廻し、えい!!バサリ――えい!!バサリ――と、何本か斬り、その中の一本をつて、切り口を示したりした。

かくて、石嶺は、身の正當防衛を認められたばかりでなく、警察の道場へ招かれて、空術の武勇を演じ、時々は、その講習などもするようになつたという。

Karate
A Story From the Venerable Karate Authority Funakoshi Gichin

There was a man named Sekiryo[116] who lived in Yawakawa, a village known for its paper making industry in Shuri. One day he was working at a farming village. He had wrapped up his work and was readying to head home when some farmhands began to shout all sorts of things at him, clearly looking for a fight. Sekiryo endured their insults but instead of reacting, simply picked up his tools and started walking home. However, the farmhands were persistent and surrounded Sekiryo and began shoving him about.

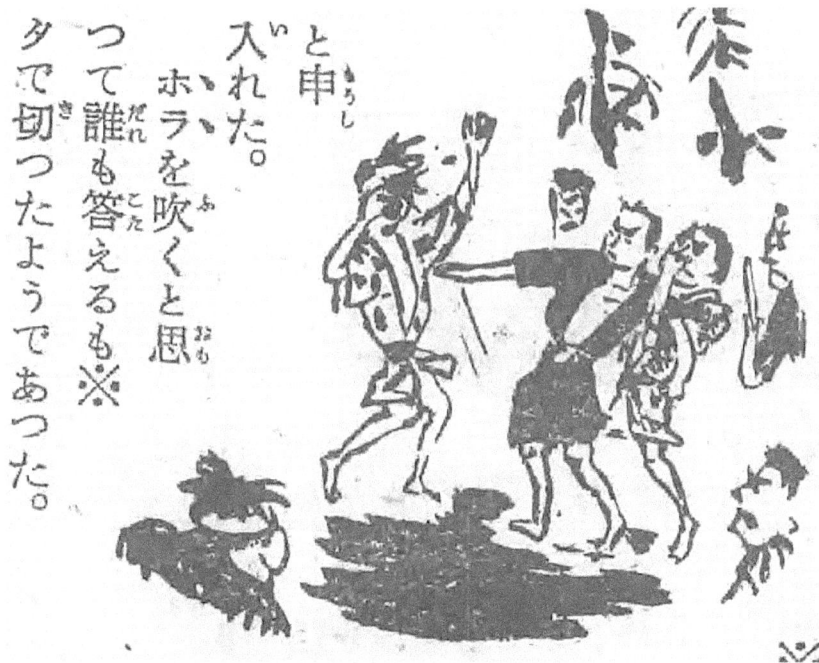

Finally, Seikiryo had had enough. He swung his right hand out in a sweeping motion which caught one of the men in the forehead, slicing him open. With that, everyone erupted in panic, shouting, "This guy has some kind of blade!" Eventually a patrolman from a police substation arrived and slapped handcuffs on Sekiryo, before hauling him off.

---

[116] Also read as "Ishimine" however this book lists it as Sekiryo.

沖縄縣で空手術が盛んになったのは、多分その頃からの事で、石嶺が有名になる頃は、それ程盛んとはいえなかった。

石鎖は『えい!!』という氣合いもろとも、天井に平べつたく吸いついたり、手がかりも足がかりもない石垣塀を『やつ!!』という掛声とともに、ヤモリか飛鳥のように、横這いしてみせたりした。しかし、上には上がいる。

更に彼より五十年程遡れば、『眞壁のチヤーン』とか『牧志』という人がいて、これは人間というよりも、烏か天狗の類で『えい!!』というと、首里城の犬手にある二重櫓の中山門にとび上つたり※、※その軒にぶら下つたり、丈餘の石垣をとび越したりまるで超人的だつたそうである。そういう人達でも、人に接する時は、まるで氣の弱い人のようであつたといわれている。

つまり空手は平和の技であって、保身の術以外の何物でもないのである。

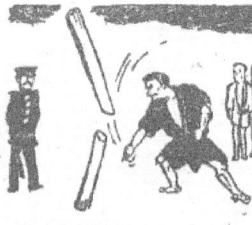

（四方山三郎）

No matter how much Sekiryo explained that it was a proper case of self-defense, the police refused to believe him. Looking out the window of the police station he noticed some pieces of abandoned trellis in the garden. He asked someone to fetch him one of the poles, which were round pieces of wood and about 2 Sun, 2 inches/6 centimeters, in diameter and about 2 Ken, 14 feet/3.6 meters.
"Please watch how I cut this with my bare hands! If you would like a particular length, just say the word!"
None of the assembled officers said anything as they were sure that he was just bragging.

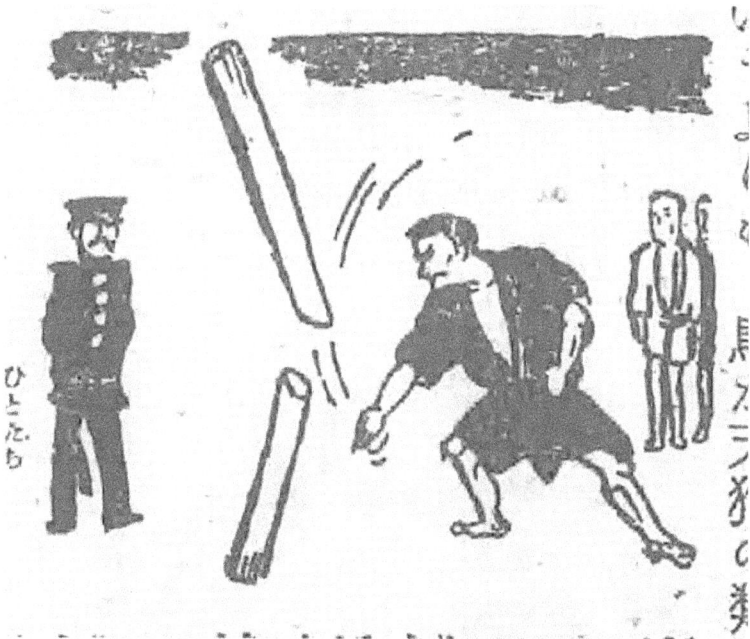

Then, with a shout of *Ei!* he sliced the bottom two feet off the pole. The cut end looked like it had been cut with an extremely sharp Nata. At that moment everyone shouted *Ah!* in shock and surprise.
"Please feel free to state which length of pole you would like!"
He went around and cut a piece for each officer with a *Ei!* Chop! *Ei* Chop! Showing each the officer the cut end of the pole.

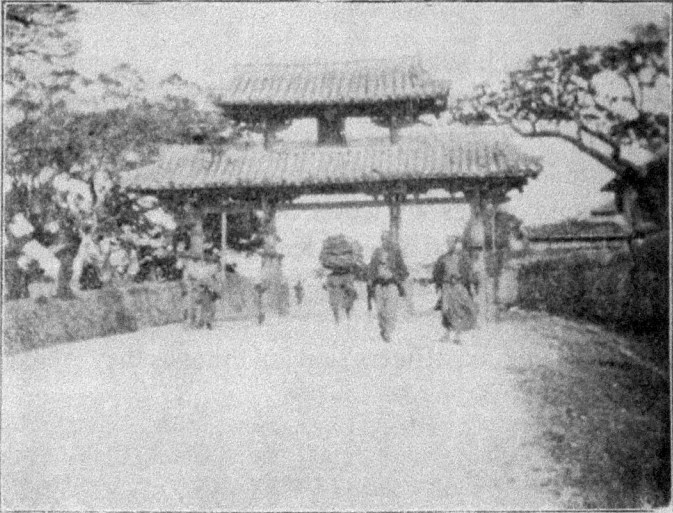

The Gateway of Propriety.

Chuzan Middle Mountain Gate in front of Shuri Castle
The original was torn down due to decay in 1908
Life in the Luchu Islands by Furness, William Henry 1899

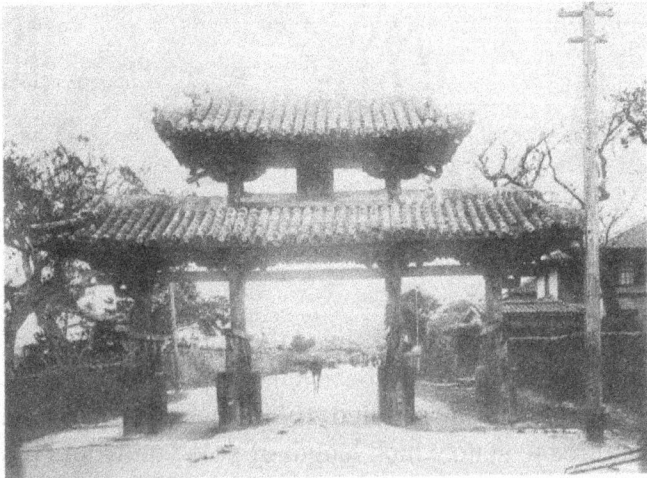

※旧首里城に登って行く途中にあった中山門（俗称・綾城―アヤジョウ―又は下の鳥井―シムントイ）。

Nostalgic Okinawa 望郷沖縄 1901

In the end Sekiryo was not only able to prove he only acted in self-defense, but he was also invited to the police Dojo to demonstrate the powerful martial art of Karate Jutsu. This eventually led him to occasionally teaching courses in Karate at the police station.

It seems likely that Karate Jutsu began to become popular in Okinawa prefecture around this time. Karate was not particularly popular until Sekiryo became famous.

Sekiryo would shout *Ei!* and cling flat to the ceiling. With a shout of *Ya!* he would leap on a stone wall that seemingly had no place to grip with either hands or feet. Despite this he would crawl across it like a gecko or flit across it like a bird going ever higher and higher.

If you go back fifty years you will encounter men like Makabe no Chyan and Bokushi. To say they are men is probably a mistake they are more akin to birds or Tengu, mountain goblins. With a shout of *Ei!* they would leap up onto the Chuzan Gate in front of Shuri Castle and hang from the rafters. Or they would leap over ten-foot stone walls and other such feats that leave you with the feeling they are superhuman. Despite this, when people who have met them described these men, they said they were gentle almost to the point of being timid.

In other words, Karate is a peaceful technique. It is nothing more than a method of self-defense.

Yomiuri Newspaper
June 29th 1952

Smashing ten roof tiles with one violent strike
Demonstrate celebrating the opening of a Dojo

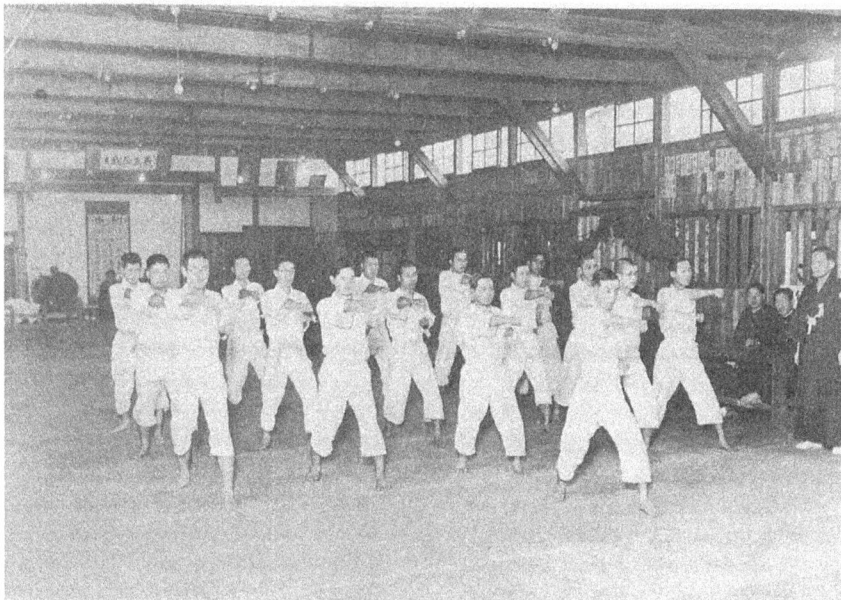

Karate Rank Test at Nodai University, 1936
Judo Kendo Dojo

Yomiuri Newspaper
June 29th 1952

Smashing ten roof tiles with one violent strike
Demonstrate celebrating the opening of a Dojo

Starting at 5:00 PM on the 28th in Chuo Ward Tsukiji Nicchome, at a certain construction company a Karate Dojo opening ceremony was held. The owner of the Dojo is President Tanaka Kiyogen who used to be a member of the Communist Party. The instructor is the founder of Wado School Karate Jutsu Otsuka Hironori (59 years old.)

University students from Tokyo, Meiji, Nichidai, Nodai and other universities stacked up 10 wooden boards or 10 roof tiles until they were nearly a foot tall and cracked them in half with one blow from their fists, feet or head. There was much applause in response to this. Recently there has been a surge in people looking to study Karate, and those with no experience are invited to join.

Picture is from Dojo opening

Funakoshi Yoshinori
Senior Instructor, Japan Karate Organization
Asahi Newspaper
April 27ᵗʰ 1957

船越　義珍（よしのり）氏（日本空手協会最高師範）二十六日午前八時四十五分老肺のため東京都文京区駒込林町七の自宅で死去。八十六。告別式は五月十日午後二時から東京雑司ヶ谷の祖蔡堂で。日本空手道の創始者として慶大、東大、早大など各大学の師範として空手の普及に尽した。

Funakoshi Yoshinori[117]
Senior Instructor, Japan Karate Organization

Funakoshi died on the 26th of April at 8:45 in the morning of elderly lungs at Tokyo at his house in Number Seven, Komagome Hayashi Cho, Bunkyo Ward Tokyo. He was eighty-six. His funeral will be at Soshigaya Funeral Home on May 10th at 2pm.

Funakoshi was the founder of Japan Karaedo and served as a Karate instructor, and succeeded in expanding the art to Keio, Tokyo, Waseda and other universities.

---

[117] Yoshinori is a more "Japanese" style of reading the name Gichin. Reading the name as "Gichin" has a decidedly Chinese characteristic, and Funakoshi may have used this reading on mainland Japan. Though it is possible it is an editorial mistake.

Meisho Juku
明正塾
Dormitory for Students From Okinawa

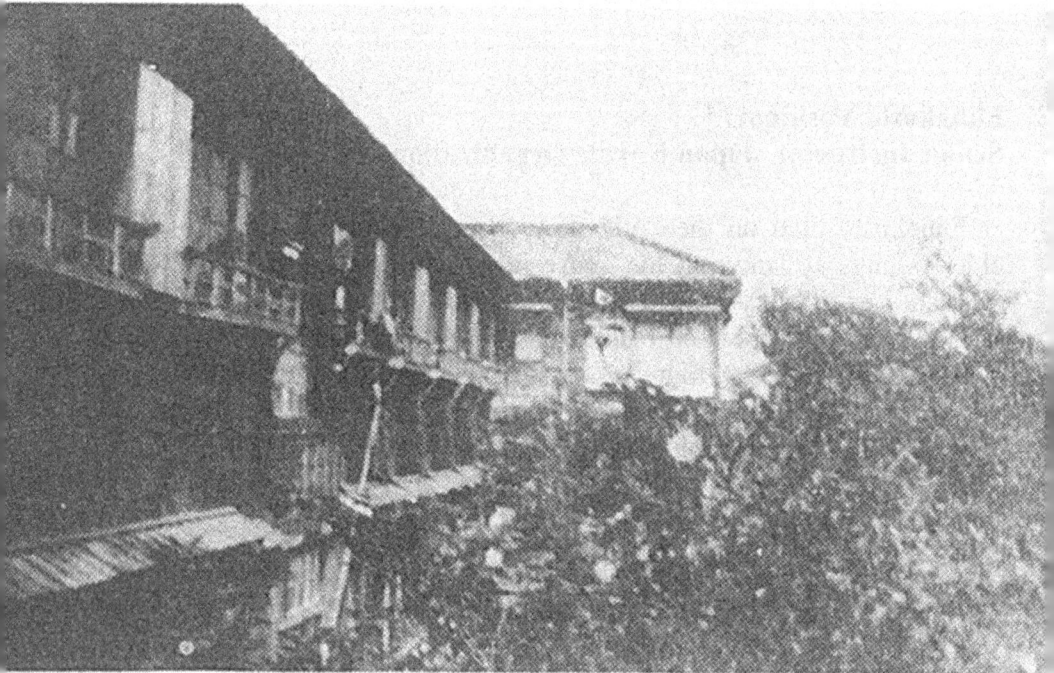

The Meisho Juku in Taisho 11 (1922)

When Funakoshi Gichin travelled to Mainland Japan in 1921, to attend the First National Athletic Exhibition, he initially stayed at a Ryokan inn, however since his stay was extended by requests for more demonstrations, he ended up moving to the Meisho Juku, a dormitory for students from Okinawa. Gima Shinkin and Fujiwara Ryozo discuss this era in *A Conversation About Recent Karatedo History,*

Gima Shinkin[118]

Funakoshi Gichin Shihan's primary objective when going to Tokyo was to participate in the First National Athletic Exhibition and he had every intention of returning home after it finished. He had no plan to live in Tokyo when he travelled there. Kano Jigoro Kancho and Kaneshiro Saburo Sensei were both aware of this. That being said, he was asked, "Would you be willing to delay your return to your hometown in Okinawa for three days and do a demonstration of Karate Jutsu?"

At the lunch following the Athletic Exhibition, Kano Jigoro said,

I had been planning to go on a business trip to China however, even if I change my plans, Mr. Funakoshi will soon, unfortunately, be returning to Okinawa, so I was wondering if it would be possible for young Mr. Gima to come to our Dojo and teach us some Karate Jutsu Kata?

Obviously, Kano Sensei was making the proposal with the understanding that Funakoshi Sensei would be returning home. However, at that time, as was more or less commonly known, I was only really adept at Naihanchi. Kano Jigoro said to me,

Young Gima you are a student so you are no doubt overjoyed about your summer vacation. While you may well have plans for the summer, if not, would you be willing to use your summer vacation to teach us some Karate Jutsu Kata?

---

[118] Gima Shinkin　儀間真謹　(1896~1989)
Fujiwara Ryozo　藤原稜三　(1925~?)

Later, when Funakoshi Shihan delayed his return to Okinawa, I ended up being released from the responsibility of leading the demonstration.

Fujiwara

However, according to Kano Jigoro's diary, he did in fact travel to China. So, you didn't end up using your summer vacation to teach a seminar?

Gima

Well, that is more or less true. However, while Kano Jigoro was away in China, our plan to have a demonstration at the Kodokan Dojo appeared in the newspapers. Former Admiral Yashiro Rokuro saw the article and he, among others, began to inquire about Karate demonstrations. In the end, Funakoshi Shihan and I went to the Yagyu Heikikyo Kan, Nikaido Taiso Juku, Sho Tai's residence and other places and conducted demonstrations introducing Karate Jutsu while we waited for Kano Jigoro to return. Thus, my last summer vacation was spent doing Karate Jutsu Enbu.

Funakoshi Shihan had delayed his return first by a week, then by two and he spent the time making connections all over mainland Japan. So, though we wanted to get Kano's thoughts on the matter of Karate, we ended up having to wait for Kano Jigoro to return from abroad before we could find out. I would like to note that the honorarium we received for conducting the demonstrations did not amount to a lot of money and by August we were out of funds, as the amount we received was like "sparrow's tears," a pittance. Thus, we were forced to settle our bill at the Ryokan inn and move into the Meisho Juku Dormitory.

Fujiwara

Kano Jigoro Kancho was very interested in Karate Jutsu, wasn't he?

Gima

Yes, he was very enthusiastic about it. You can clearly see this if you read the book *National Exercise Techniques for Mutual*

Prosperity of Yourself and Others[119] that Kano Jigoro Sensei wrote. You can see the great influence Karate had in the Kata he included.

-A Conversation About Recent Karatedo History
近代空手道の歴史を語る：対談
1986

Another person familiar with the Meisho Juku dormitory was Miyajima Chojun.[120] Miyajima was a famous educator born in Naha who enrolled in Toyo University in Tokyo. While attending class he stayed as Meisho Juku dormitory and trained with Funakoshi Gichin.

Meisho Juku was built between the end of the Meiji era and the beginning of the Taisho Era.[121] It was a dormitory for students born in Okinawa Prefecture built by Okinawa Prefecture. There was a courtyard in the center where Sakura trees grew, and in the spring they would bloom wonderfully. Kamiyama Seiryo Sensei was the principle of the Academy.[122] Kamiyama Sensei was our great Senpai who built the Academy for Okinawa. Sensei's office had a three-meter-long bookshelf packed with Western books. His wife told me that even if he got home late, he would always read for at least two hours.

-Miyajima Chojun
The Story of Miyajima Chojun 伝宮島長純
1981

Miyajima also describes the Meisho Juku training space, the students and Funakoshi Sense's training philosophy.

There was a four-Tatami mat room to the side of the entrance to the dormitory where Funakoshi Gichin Sensei would teach

---

[119] 精力善用国民体育 1924

[120] 宮島長純 (1906-?)

[121] The Meiji era ended in 1912, which was followed by the Taisho era, which lasted until 1926.

[122] 神山 政良 (1882~1978) Born into a Samurai family in Shuri, he later attended Oxford University. His wife, Yaeko, was the daughter of Sho Tai, the final king of Ryukyu.

Karate. There fourteen or fifteen beautiful college girls majoring in medicine and dentistry taking lessons. I had reached a level where I tied a black belt around my uniform so Sensei allowed me to enter the instruction room. The dormitory students were not allowed into the instruction room while Karate instruction was taking place. The others were very jealous that I was the only one allowed in the room when training was going on.
He taught by saying,

In spring the Sakura bloom, in fall we can enjoy the leaves changing color. Similarly, in Karate the left and right hands repeat the same technique.

I was always there asking Funakoshi Sensei questions.
-Miyajima Chojun

Miyajima also described a curious incident at the dormitory, involving Funakoshi Gichin.

At the time, only those registered at the dormitory could stay the night there. However, a youth named Yamanokuchi [123] never seemed to go home. Even when someone told him the rule was, he had to go home, Yamanokuchi would simply reply, "Oh, really?" and the next morning we would find him sleeping in the common bedroom.
One day there was an incident. Takaesu, who was featured in Hirotsu Kazuo's story, *Wandering Ryukyu Man*, walked into the Meisho Juku dormitory after he had been drinking Sake. [124] After asking if Funakoshi Sensei was in, he walked into Sensei's office and yanked a Rokushaku Bo off the wall and began threatening everybody with it. This threw the students into a panic and they began to flee while shouting, "What's he doing? What's he doing?"

---

[123] Yamanokuchi Baku 山之口 貘 (1903~1963) Born in Naha, he moved to Tokyo in 1922 at the age of 19 to attend art school but quit after a month.
[124] Hirotsu Kazuo 広津和郎 (1891~1968) Born in Tokyo, Hirotsu was a novelist and translator.

Suddenly, he went into the kitchen and grabbed a knife and began swinging it around. The whole dormitory erupted in panic.

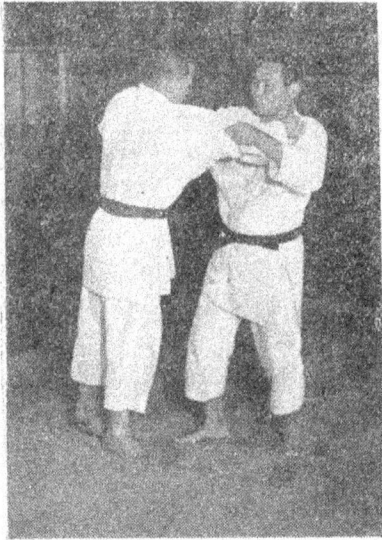 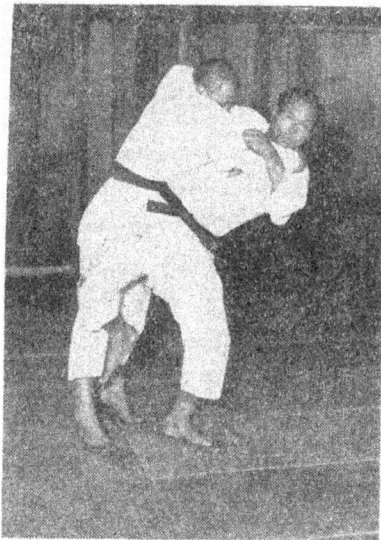

(第 一 圖)   (第 二 圖)

Hane Goshi Spring hip throw steps one and two
Judo Magazine April 1940

A patrolman who was walking by the front gate heard the commotion and rushed in. He soaked a towel in water and charged Takaesu before the man knew what was happening. The patrolman swung the towel, aiming for the knife in Takaesu's hand. Next, the patrolman toppled him with Hane Goshi and put his right arm in an armbar before dragging him out the front door and down onto the dirt floor of the entrance chamber.

一本背負の方法

日本教育柔道要義

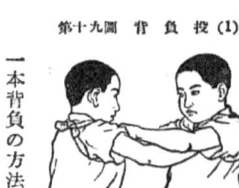

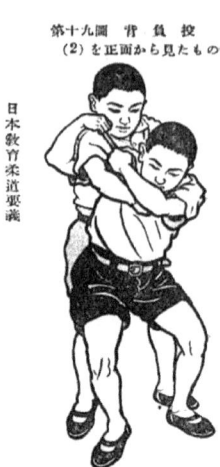

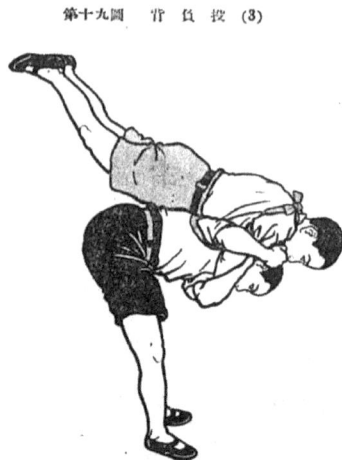

Seoi Nage steps one through three
Outline of the Japanese Physical Education Judo Program
日本教育柔道要義 1940 By Sakuraba Takeshi 桜庭武 1892-1941

The patrolman then threw him with a powerful Seoi Nage. The officer was able to subdue the man quickly with his rapid application of well-rehearsed technique. In the next moment he was applying the Tenawa, rope handcuffs. In the following days, Takaesu surprised everyone by claiming that, "Meisho Juku is a dangerous place!"

When the commander of the patrol squad arrived on the scene, he was quite critical,

If you can't handle one drunken lout then maybe you should take down your sign calling yourself a Karate instructor!

However, Funakoshi Sensei replied quietly,

Since he was from our hometown island, we tried to restrain him in a calmer manner.

In response the commander said,

How on earth do you confront a man with a knife in a calm manner?!

With that he yanked Takaesu roughly up and hauled him off to the station.

-Miyajima Chojun
The Story of Miyajima Chojun 伝宮島長純
1981

Regarding how police used rope before handcuffs to arrest suspects, the 1941 book *How to Arrest Suspects* 逮捕の要領 shows how rope handcuffs were used to restrain suspects.

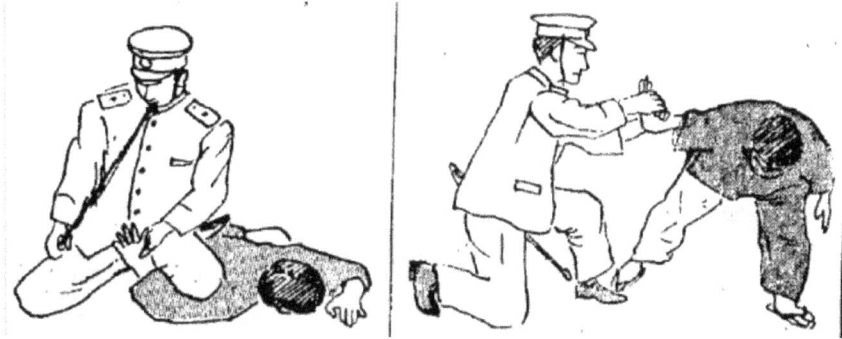

As the illustration on the right shows, reverse the attacker's wrist upward until he falls on his right shoulder. As you pull him down, plant your left knee on top of his upper arm to control it. Then twist his right hand behind his back before rapidly using your police rope to tie him up.

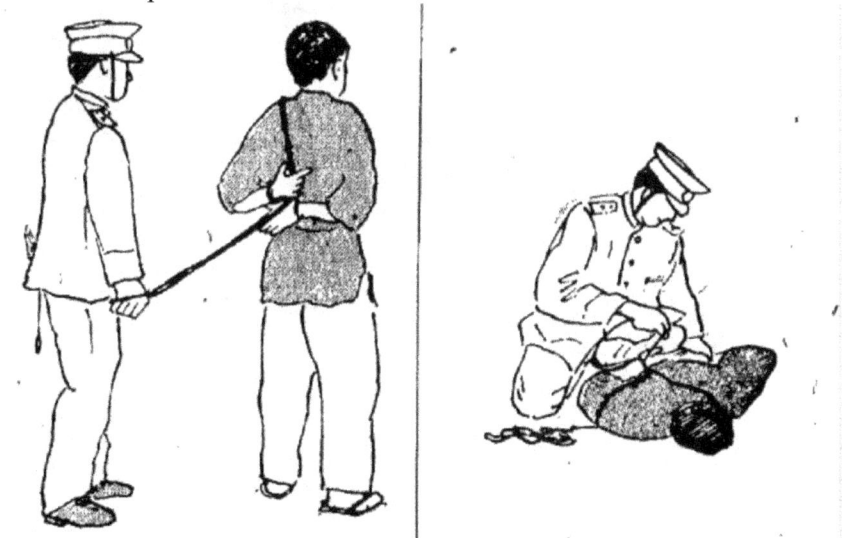

After tying off his right wrist, thereby gaining control of it, pass the rope over his left shoulder and under his right armpit. Then wrap the rope around his right wrist again before bending his left arm behind his back and tying it above his right hand.

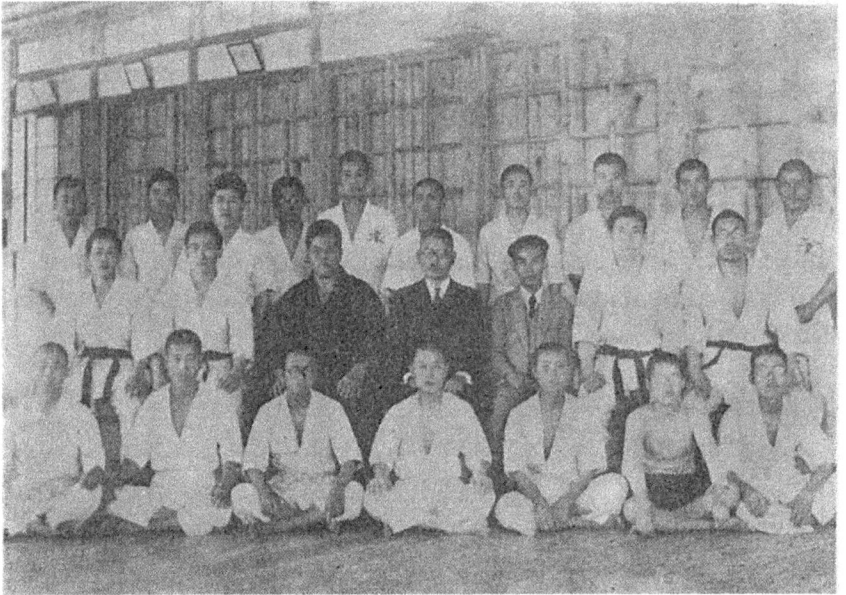

Miyagi Chojun 宮城長順 (1888 ~ 1953) with the Naha City School
of Commerce Karate Team circa 1937.

Miyajima describes Takaesu encountering Funakoshi Gichin in the course of his rampage.

> When Takaesu was thrashing about with the Rokushaku Bo, Funakoshi Sensei was walking quietly down the hallway. Takaesu, moving up behind Sensei, began attacking with the Bo. Funakoshi did not turn around but continued walking calmly down the hallway. When Takaesu struck left, Sensei blocked with his left hand. When Takaesu struck right, Sensei blocked with this right hand, all without turning around.
>
> To be able to defend against strikes from a Rokushaku Bo from behind without turning around is an example of the ultimate in martial arts.

-Miyajima Chojun
The Story of Miyajima Chojun 伝宮島長純

Miyajima also interacted with other famous Karate practitioners. After he became a teacher, he was assigned to Naha City School of Commerce[125] in Showa 12 (1937.) Once there he was put in charge of the Karate Club. The Karate team instructor was Miyagi Chojun, founder of the Goju School of Karate.

At the School of Commerce 20% of the physical education score was based on students' performance in Karate. The club often did Karate demonstrations for visiting groups which were very well received.

---

[125] Naha City School of Commerce 那覇市商業学校

www.ingramcontent.com/pod-product-compliance
Lightning Source LLC
Chambersburg PA
CBHW070838300326
41935CB00038B/1134